The Secret World of Microbes

The Good, the Bad and the Ugly

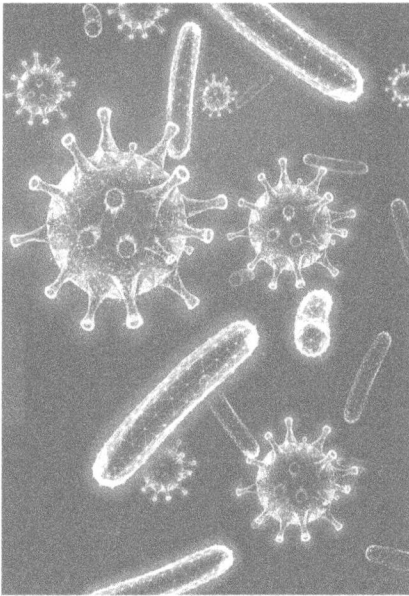

Dr. Rajkumar Chetty
MBBS MD FRCPath

The Secret World of Microbes: The Good, the Bad and the Ugly

Other books by Dr. Rajkumar Chetty

The Myth of the Economy: What Can Nature Teach us That Harvard Does Not
A Unified Theory of Human Disease: Is Information Failure the Basis for all
Diseases?
The Puppet Show: How Organisms Dance to the Tune of the Environment
God Molecules: The Biochemistry of God
The Myth of Information Technology: Amazing Wonders of Biological
Communication
The Myth of Human Intelligence: Nature's Incredible ways of Problem-Solving
The Universe as a Complex System: What Can Modern Science and Eastern
Philosophy tell us about Order, Creation, God and Religion?

© 2023 Dr. Rajkumar Chetty
Print ISBN ISBN 978-1-960405-21-0
ebook ISBN 978-1-960405-22-7

Cover Design by Guy D. Corp
www.GrafixCorp.com

STAIRWAY PRESS—APACHE JUNCTION

STAIRWAY⹀PRESS

www.StairwayPress.com
1000 West Apache Trail
Suite 126
Apache Junction, AZ 85120 USA

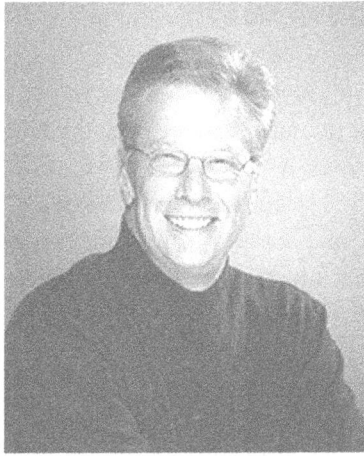

Forward

VIRUSES LIVE TO mutate. But as Dr. Chetty correctly points out in this entertaining, thought-provoking volume on the secret world of microbes, "Viruses are the most populous of all creatures on Planet Earth and do not even figure in the classification scheme of life."

What?

That's right, a virus isn't considered a living organism. Why? Because they lack the metabolic factory necessary to be classified as such.

So, to be more precise, I'll amend my statement to: Viruses *exist* to mutate. And, by the way, so do other microbes. Cases in point: the Omicron variant of the SARS-CoV-2 virus and the Methicillin resistant strain of Staphylococcus Aureus. They've evolved because of the constant Darwinian struggle we health professionals create for them: MRSA (Methicillin-Resistant Staphylococcus Aureus) is a prime example of a resistant strain of bacteria created by us doctors.

But not all microbes are bad guys. Numerous bacteria live symbiotically with us in our gut and on our skin, for example.

And when they do, our bodies turn a blind eye to them. Why do some bacteria help us digest food and sustain our bodies, while others prevent our lungs from exchanging oxygen? From the perspective of our immune system, what's the difference between the good and the bad guys? How does it know the difference?

Why does the chickenpox virus lie dormant in our body for years only to become symptomatic Shingles decades later? Why can a Streptococci infection damage the heart or kidneys years after the infection was eradicated? Why do some viruses—such as the hepatitis virus—target only one specific organ?

We also are shown how the study of virology has started spinning off innovative gene editing approaches for treating genetically based diseases like Cystic Fibrosis.

In this book, Dr. Chetty successfully weaves philosophy and biology into intriguing questions and answers about the microbial environment in which we all live.

—Allen Wyler, MD

Allen Wyler is an author and retired neurosurgeon who lives in Seattle.

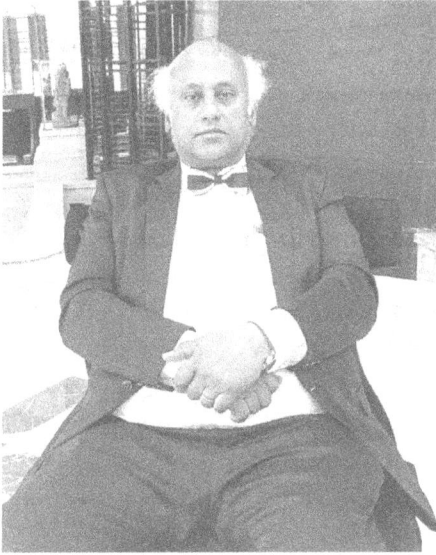

About Dr. Chetty

DR. RAJKUMAR CHETTY is an Indian-British medical doctor. After completing his medical education, he specialized in Clinical Biochemistry and Pharmaceutical Medicine and currently works as the Head of Medical Laboratory Services at a hospital in Dubai.

He is a Fellow of the Royal College of Pathologists, United Kingdom. Dr. Chetty is also a Fellow of the Faculty of the Pharmaceutical Medicine, The Royal College of Physicians, UK. He has worked for the National Health Service UK for many years as a Chemical Pathologist. He spent over seven years working in Pharmaceutical R&D at the global pharmaceutical company AstraZeneca at their Alderley Park research facility near Manchester. During this time, he was involved in many clinical trials of new drugs as a Principal Investigator.

Dr. Chetty is registered with the General Medical Council

UK as a specialist in two medical specialties—Clinical Biochemistry and Pharmaceutical medicine. In total he has more than 35 years of professional experience in hospital practice, teaching, and research gained in India, United Kingdom, Saudi Arabia, and UAE.

Dr. Chetty has a deep-rooted interest in scientific philosophy and revels in thinking, writing and talking about profound worldly phenomena and their scientific basis. In terms of writing experience Dr. Chetty has published five books in his native language of Tamil on the topic of scientific basis of spirituality. He has also published seven eBooks in English on a variety of topics touching upon spiritualism, economics, Information science, medicine and philosophy.

Three more of his works are awaiting publication.

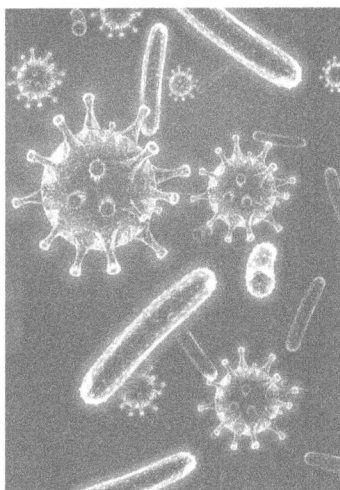

Chapter 1

WHOM TO BLAME FOR THE GLOBAL VIRUS MANIA?

THERE HAS BEEN mass hysteria since the Corona virus outbreak happened a few years ago. People are very scared. They fear losing their lives. They fear economic harm. The Corona virus, though infinitely small, dealt a death blow from which humanity has not recovered. Goliath beat David black and blue.

How did this happen?

There has never been a time when the average public were so involved in science. Things changed. Many became experts in virology. We all now know much about gene mutations, viral variants, vaccines and whatnot.

Viruses became newsworthy—attracting the same level of interest normally reserved for celebrities, musicians, athletes and cinema. A new viral variant seen in one corner of the globe is enough to cause massive depression and fear amongst all homo sapiens. We are that scared.

This book addresses the world of microbes—not just the Corona Virus. There is a vast, secret world where microbes thrive about which we know very little and have never shown any interest in knowing more, until the Corona virus struck.

Now, we are all ears when someone says something about viruses or microbes in general. The Corona virus earned a huge respect not just for itself, but for the entire microbial kind.

In this book, I show that microbes come in three types: the good, bad and ugly. We always focus on the bad and ugly types, but never care to think that there is a whole lot of good brought about by the microbes on our planet.

Are microbes always villains? Are they always a nuisance? The answer is a resounding no. That is what this book talks about.

The whole world was in a panic mode for the past few years. This level of panic was unprecedented. We have not seen anything like this in our lifetime. No one would have even dreamt that airports worldwide would be shut down with all aircraft parked there unused. This was unbelievable.

News of Corona was everywhere. Turn on the TV and there was nothing other than Corona news, death statistics and updates about the vaccine. Open a newspaper and the whole newspaper had nothing other than Corona.

Corona gripped the entire world. Homo sapiens who planned to create future settlements on Mars would have loved to be able to do so, because the planet Earth was on lockdown.

Countries with nuclear arsenals that can decimate humanity in a flash succumbed to a tiny, invisible virus.

What happened to create this level of scare? Haven't we seen viral pandemics before—other pathogenic outbreaks like Cholera, Plague etc.? Why did we freak out this time? Is the real threat the Corona virus or was the panic a side-effect of social media influence?

Did we suffer because we humans failed to sufficiently look out for microbes? Could we have done better if we had cooperated to study and catalogue all viruses and bacteria rather than spending our money and resources on fighting each other?

We spend more money on wars against our own humanity than on finding cures for microbes. How much funding has been given to universities for microbial research and how much did we spend on meaningless, egoistic wars?

Did we get beat by the virus in our own garden while we were meaninglessly looking out at galaxies and stars so far away? Or, when we were busy fighting each other?

There are 200 known viruses that can harm mankind. SARS, MERS, Influenza, Ebola, Marburg, Hanta, Zika, Nipah and the list goes on. So far, we have documented about 6,500 types of viruses in the world—of which 200 are capable of infecting man. The rest do not bother us. It is estimated that the total number of viruses on the planet is likely upwards of three-hundred-thousand, and this is more of a guesstimate. Some say it could be even more.

In the past, did we make any attempt to know about all these viruses? Then we have no moral right to grieve the devastation of the global economy caused by a virus that could have been eliminated if there had been global research on biological threats in nature.

It is said that it would cost 2-6 billion dollars to conduct a thorough cataloguing of all the viruses that exist on the planet. Considering the meaningless spending of money and resources on anti-human wars and the pilferage of money in corrupt political circles—not to mention the bad planning and waste of resources at national levels, it is very easy to grasp the idea that these 2-6 billion dollars are worth investment that could have saved the trillions lost due to the lockdown.

If all countries agreed to share the cost, it would be so easy. Why hasn't our society done this? Is it because there are no profit-making possibilities? If there was direct money-making potential in this exercise, multinational corporations would fall over each other to do this. National governments would back them and the banks would fund them. The lack of foresight and wisdom caused losses to the tune of trillions of dollars and a few million human lives.

Who is to be blamed?

The finger points right at us.

I have no doubt we failed to take preventive measures. Now

we run from pillar to post trying to develop a vaccine for the Corona virus. All the time, the lame excuse is put forward that it is difficult to find a vaccine for viruses because they mutate all the time—which is like a moving target.

That is why we are unable to shoot them down with a vaccine. I have two questions. We had two other viruses (SARS-2009, and MERS- COV) hit us in the last 10 years. They belong to the same Corona virus family. They had at least some features that resemble their brother COVID-19 virus.

Why did we not bother to develop a vaccine based on this information? Are we now paying the price for our callousness? The second question is why we had good vaccines for smallpox, polio, measles, mumps, etc.? Why do we look at the external coat of the virus for choosing our target? Why can't we look at the internal structure, or process of the virus, which is not known to mutate at all? Are we so intellectually lazy that we never bothered to do this?

A glaring truth about the impotency of human race against these invisible viral enemies is that we never succeeded in finding drugs against them and that includes the common cold virus too!

Don't you think it is paradoxical that we claim to have advanced so much in the medical sciences, but we do not have any medicines for viruses? What is the problem? Is the virus too powerful or did we lack the motivation to find suitable anti-viral medicines until we got hit badly.

Treatment for the AIDS virus may be a small exception, but why haven't we shown the same level of resolve against so many other disease-causing viruses? One reason could be that most viruses are self-limiting—after a period of illness, they burn out.

We realized this and decided to take a casual approach. The AIDS virus gave us a jolt in the mid-1980s and is still a killer. The other factor spurring us into action was it caused an inconvenience because it interfered with our personal lives.

For man, that was enough reason to go all out and find a cure for it. Having said that, have we really succeeded in the fight against the AIDS virus?

I am unable to say 'yes.'

We managed to delay death, but I do not think we really found cures that will help us evade death due to the AIDS virus. The AIDS virus continues to kill 1-2 million people every year since the 1980s and that death rate seems even more than the current COVID death rate! Do we really want to boast that we have cured AIDS?

7.8 billion plus people on this planet cursed the Corona virus. It messed with everyone's life. Humanity is scared to death of the Corona virus. This may be the result of the impact of social media where something unworthy got such wide publicity. A virus with only 2-3% mortality is dreaded like we have never encountered any other pathogen before in our lives! People worried, maybe, thinking it is going to be deadly like the Spanish Flu that hit us early 20th Century.

The real reason is that there was no effective medicine known for Corona virus. Until now, little did we care to think there has never been any medicine for any virus.

Why did we panic only for Corona?

This applies to the common cold virus too. Why did we freak out about the Corona—putting our national economies in the ICU by locking nations down!

It is said that all over the world, 5,000 people die every day from TB. This is the global death rate for Corona virus since it struck us in December 2019. Why did we panic so much about Corona, but not for the TB bacterium? This is very strange. Interestingly, both these crooks target our lungs.

At any given moment, there are at least 10 million people with full blown TB. Whether you believe it or not, one in three people on this planet are already infected by the TB bacteria.

But the infected do not cause blatant disease. Such patients are like asymptomatic carriers of the COVID virus. In the case of TB, such asymptomatic carriers are said to be affected by a latent infection. About 10% of these people will develop full blown disease at some point in time. The 5,000 people who die of TB everyday amount to almost 2 million deaths a year. This is much more than the current COVID death figures. Nobody seems to panic about TB as much as they do about COVID.

Why is this so?

Is it because TB affects mostly underdeveloped countries? Or is it because it has been here for centuries, and we accept it as a way of life? Or is it because TB established itself as a regular culprit a long time before these media frenzies existed? Did we get used to this menace? Is that why we learned to live with it? Is that what will happen with Corona too?

It is possible that Corona will never go away and continue to kill us at some steady rate, and we will accept it as part of our lives. Even today, the regular Flu virus kills an estimated 500,000 to 600,000 people all over the world which works out to almost 1,800 deaths every day. This information comes to us from statistics released by the Centers for Disease Control (CDC) in the US.

We just carry on.

Just like that, maybe we will also carry on with Corona.

I believe COVID-19 gained unprecedented prominence in human history due to social media. Even when its cousin, SARS-2009, came around, social media platforms were not as powerful as they are today. We receive tens of messages every day saying mundane things like 'Good morning.' We want more firepower in our messages.

The COVID virus was an automatic fit for a gory tale. Everyone wants to hear such stories. More than anything, lack of effective treatment caught people's attention. Before, nobody cared that there was no effective treatment for viruses. That did not bother them. Social media overplayed the threat like all the newspapers do. The point that the COVID virus kills only 2-3% of the infected people was ignored because it would dilute the impact of the story.

The power of WhatsApp and Facebook grew so much that it only takes milliseconds for a message to spread all over the world. This helped all planetary inhabitants worry together. The mania reached such heights that some people even committed suicide once diagnosed positive with COVID-19!

In some countries like India, whole families of an infected person were treated like lepers. There were public protests trying to prevent dead patient's bodies from being buried in cemeteries nearer to their homes!

Day by day, the extent of public mania reached greater heights. Nowadays there are many products sold in the shops with the tag anti-viral. Anti-viral masks, anti-viral plywood and anti-viral soap and so on! The word anti-viral is the fashion of the day and marketers—as always—latch onto this for making money.

Masks now come from designer shops! One product I saw recently was a nice, compact, flat box meant for carrying masks.

The Corona virus infiltrated every walk of our lives.

One can confidently say that the same Corona virus outbreak would have had far less impact if it had happened 15 years ago or earlier.

We would have worried less then.

We would not have had WhatsApp, YouTube, and Facebook to feed fear. MERS-CoV and SARS were all similar outbreaks that happened around 15 years ago, and they were all cousins to the COVID-19 virus because they all belonged to the same family. Why didn't we react to these outbreaks as we did to COVID-19?

One of the little-known facts about COVID-19 mortality is that the cause of the death is not the viral damage. What kills? It is the immune attack against the virus that turns against your own body.

Doctors call this the Cytokine storm.

Cytokines are protective agents released by our immune system. They are targeted against the infecting microbe. They are supposed to attack microbes and help us to escape microbial diseases. What happens in some individuals is that the immune system overreacts, presumably because of genetically determined differences, and produces an excessive number of Cytokines.

These Cytokines have systemic effects causing damage to our body. What was intended to attack the microbe ends up causing a lot of collateral damage and ultimately death. I suppose this is like what we see in wars. Bombs and other weapons used against each other were meant to kill the soldiers. But we see civilian damage and civilian deaths as well.

I liken the Cytokine storm to our lockdowns. Both are excessive, unwarranted reactions. In the case of the Cytokine storm, the individual human body made the mistake of overreacting to the microbe and met its demise due to collateral damage, which due to ignorance, we blamed on the virus.

Lockdown, which caused untold economic damage to all countries in the world, was an unreasonable, unwanted, excessive political reaction to a microbe.

The lockdown killed our societies, not the virus. I feel that the fear mongering—fueled by social media—forced governments to overreact because they thought inaction amidst global fear would be construed as governmental failure. The price countries paid for this misguided decision could haunt us for decades.

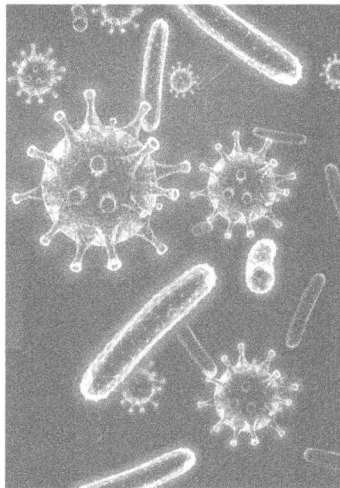

Chapter 2

DAVID versus GOLIATH—WHY IS GOLIATH LOSING?

THE CORONA VIRUS waged war against humanity. Wars have been commonplace throughout history. When one country invades another, there is a motif behind it. It could be the greed for power, or the desire to loot the wealth of that nation, or some enmity based on a past event.

But what does this tiny virus gain by fighting us? The strange and unbelievable thing about this outwardly unequal battle is that we ran away from the enemy and hid ourselves inside our houses. It certainly was not the tiny Corona virus that lost.

Recently I saw a news item about how China has built a missile that can be launched from a submarine. This missile has a range of 12,000 kilometers. I see this news from two angles. One, we humans have such impressive technology that can shoot a bomb over such a long distance and with such precision. But we are so powerless when it comes to handling a tiny virus that is way smaller than a speck of dust.

The second angle to this news item is that China may have found a way of finishing off the business of all the countries with one invisible bomb, the corona virus, at no cost at all! It did not have to fight bitter and protracted wars with countries and the outcome is much better.

It is said that our human bodies have about 30 trillion cells. The total population of humans on the planet is a paltry 7.8 billion. The number of corona virus particles that need to enter a human body is about 1 million for a Corona virus PCR test to register positive. That is said to be the bare minimum numbers for the virus to work on infecting the human body.

If the number of corona virus particles is less than a million, then it stands less chance of surviving in the human body and causing infection. This may be because our human immune system dealt a swift blow to these tiny numbers of the corona virus.

For the sake of an argument let us say a million of these corona viruses found their way into a human body. How on earth did the tiny army of the tiny viral soldiers manage to win against us who have almost 30 million times more cells in our body than the number of corona virus particles that invaded us?

Again, for the sake of argument, let us just count the number of cellular warriors and not the whole bodies' population. White blood cells are our body's defense forces that patrol the blood sea 24/7. When a microbe manages to find its way into the body, it is like an enemy intruding into our fortress. Our white blood cellular warriors smell the intruders and quickly launch an offensive against the microbes using high-tech biological weapons.

An infection is like colonization of our lands by the unwanted enemy. The average human being has about 20-60 billion while blood cells in his body. That is a lot of soldiers in an army. As in any national defense force consisting of Army, Navy, Air Force, Coast Guards and Marine Corps, our body defense forces are also constituted by different types of white blood cells like Neutrophils, Lymphocytes, Basophils, Eosinophils and

Monocytes. Each has its task cut out and is present in huge numbers. The guys who fight viruses like Corona are the Lymphocytes. They are incidentally the largest variety of white blood cells in sheer numbers and constitute about 40-70% of the total white blood cell count.

Despite being in such huge numbers, how did we lose against Corona? Isn't it strange that Goliath is afraid of David now? Why are we hiding?

Lymphocytes can generate molecular weaponry like Antibodies, Interleukins and Interferons that are like precision-guided missiles that target microbes. Antibodies are custom-made bombs targeted against the microbes and each antibody type is tailor-made for the type of microbe it is intended to attack.

As far as I know, I do not think we have anything equivalent of this in our real-world defenses. Whether it is a gun or a cannon, it is all the same bullet or bomb. Despite all this we fought a losing battle against the Corona virus and were afraid of the virus as if we had never experienced it before. Though our human ego would hate to admit it, we basically surrendered to the Corona virus.

What is the military strategy of the Corona virus that gave it the upper hand (at least for now)? When it comes to military strategy, it is said that there are only three types known. One is attrition where you erode the combat power of the enemy forces gradually until he becomes weak. Second is Annihilation where the focus is on immediate and swift destruction of the combat power of the enemy. Third is Exhaustion wherein an indirect approach is used to hit the enemy such that he loses the will or ability to fight. This strategy is not against the armed forces but against the things that make the enemy incapable of fighting. This could include sinking the cargo ships that bring the supplies to the enemy. In the olden days when the invading army sieges a fortress, that is exactly what happened. No supplies are allowed to enter the fort and that will slowly start affecting the ability of the soldiers inside the fort to fight.

Indirect attacks these days can also aim at weakening the

economy, attacking the command control centers rather than the armed forces itself, attacking the communication systems like hacking etc.

What strategy did Corona virus follow?

I suggest it used the third strategy. Exhaustion. It hit us at our gas supply i.e., our breathing. The human body is starved of oxygen fuel and there is no way we can run our body's essential functions, including the white blood cell armed forces, without the power of oxygen.

In economic jargon, breathing can be described as a business activity wherein the body as a business corporation imports oxygen from the atmosphere. The lungs are the ports where this import takes place. The Corona virus hits right here. It did not bother to fight any of the white cell soldiers, can you believe that? It adopts the exhaustion battle strategy.

That is why Goliath is losing.

Recently the main oil field in Saudi Arabia got hit by an enemy drone cutting Saudi Arabia's oil production by 5.6 million barrels a day—which is almost 50% of its daily output. It caused a destabilization of global financial markets and a rise in oil prices. One news writer described it as a heart attack for mankind as petroleum was so vitally important for assuring the world's energy needs.

This battle strategy is aimed at exhausting the enemy. The Corona virus did the same to Homo sapiens. It hit us at the gas fields in the lungs. We have gas reserves inside our body (i.e., oxygen) that will last only 3 minutes and it could be very easy to take us down. The surprising thing is how did the Corona virus know about it?

Does it matter which of us is greater, we or the microbes? No doubt we are greater in terms of size and abilities. We are bulky and way bigger than a microbe. But this illusion does not last long if you start looking at some numbers.

Microbes apparently constitute almost 75% of the total biomass on Earth. The word biomass refers to the weight of life systems. What would be the total bodyweight of all life systems combined? It is estimated at 550 billion tons. That is a lot of weight. It sounds to me life systems have become obese meaning we are probably far too many. Mother Earth already shows signs of distress and is unable to meet the demands of supporting 550 billion tons of living matter. The consequence of this Biomass obesity is serious and no different from our own bodily obesity.

Of the 550 billion tons of total biomass, microbes account for 400 billion tons. That is a clear majority. All multicellular life forms, including animals and plants together, weigh 150 billion tons only. That is a shame. Even more shameful is we Homo sapiens contribute only about 0.5 billion tons which is disappointing.

We are a paltry 0.1% of all living matter on the planet, but somehow manage to create an aura of greatness about ourselves. We believe we control the Earth and never neglect the opportunity to look down on other life forms as second-grade citizens. In terms of weight, microbes represent 800 times more than mankind.

The funny thing is they are so small that we cannot even see it. Really the viruses are the Goliaths and not us.

Microbes have remained unicellular while multitudes of other organisms diversified into multicellular life forms. Who is smart? Is it the microbe for remaining lean and slick, or the animals and plants for becoming bulkier and multi-skilled? When examining the business world, you find both single-operation companies and multiple-operation companies.

Small and local companies are more prevalent than multinational companies.

How large are the Corona or the Influenza viruses? If you line up 100 million, they will stretch up to 1 meter only whereas each man measures around 1.5 meters. An average human being is longer than about 150 to 200 million viruses put together.

Just to give you an idea of how small a virus is let us take another everyday example. The table salt that we use daily is ground into tiny particles so tiny that they flow like water. Each of these salt grains is 10,000 times bigger than a virus, I am told. How did we end up so afraid of these tiny creatures?

The viruses are on the top of the list of most populous

creatures on the planet. They rank number one. Just how many viruses are out there? It is said that we need to multiply 10 by 10 a total of 31 times to get the viral population (10^{31}). It will be 10 Nonillion and I am sure none of the readers will have any idea what a Nonillion is. For an average reader multiplying a small number like 10 by 10 may sound not too big. But let me warn you that if you multiplied 10 by 10 just 9 times you get 1 billion. Multiply 10 by 10 for the 10th time you get 10 billion.

On the 11th time you get 100 billion and by only the 12th time you get a trillion! Then you still have a long way to go to reach 31 times.

Do you begin to grasp the astronomical number of microbes?

National Geographic magazine carried an article that said the total number of viruses on Earth outnumbers the total number of stars in the Universe by a whopping 100 million times and believe me the number of stars in our universe is not sparse by any standard.

If you thought the bacteria, the other major class of microbes, are any fewer, then you are wrong. They are equally populous. It's a small consolation that you have to multiply 10 by 10 only 30 times (not 31 times).

Another tidbit too shocking to believe is the total length of all viruses (all types of viruses including Corona) if they were lined up sequentially. This line stretches to nearly infinity. If you rode on the crest of a light wave, it would take 100 million years to start from one end of the virus line to reach the other end.

For those who do not know how fast light travels—it is 300,000 kilometers per second—1 trillion kilometers per hour.

At this speed it takes 100 million years to reach your destination. Even a mathematical genius like Ramanujam might find it impossible to fathom this kind of distance.

If you were to travel in a car, you would not reach the other end at the Universe's end—even considering that after almost 14 billion years, the Universe shows no sign of ageing and death.

Microbes are prevalent anywhere—they are in water, air, soil and even above us in the atmosphere. Take a teaspoon of soil.

It is said to contain 1 billion bacteria. In your own human body, it is estimated that there are 1,400 types of microbial species living in it. It is surely a cosmopolitan place. The human body looks like a jungle inhabited by 1,400 types of species, each in millions, and it only goes by your name. I am not even sure if we can justify calling yourself by a single name. It is like trying to call an apartment block by your name when many others live there too.

Given the abundance of microbes, it is impossible to lock yourself down from them. We adopted a worldwide lockdown strategy to escape from the Corona. But that has no impact in preventing the spread of the Corona virus.

Viruses spread by air and can rise into the atmosphere to a height as much as 3 kilometers—then they settle on the ground.

It is estimated by Dr. Curtis Suttie at Canada's British Columbia University that about 800 million viruses settle on the ground per every square meter.

This includes all kinds of virus—including the Corona. Until they settle on the ground, they could be carried long distances in the air circulation.

Maybe that is why Corona virus—which started its journey from Wuhan, China—found its way into more than 150 countries in a matter of months.

We'd have to escape to Mars to make ourselves safe from microbes. What we need is lockdown of the Earth itself.

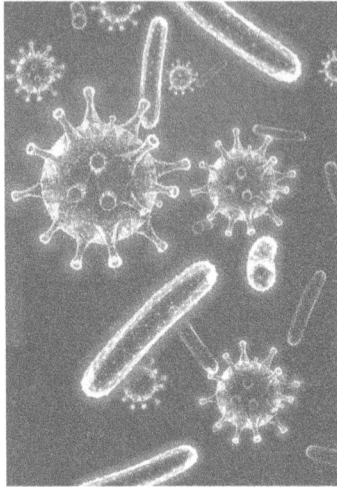

Chapter 3

MAN-MICROBE RELATIONS

OUR RELATIONSHIP WITH microbes is variable. We live in peace with some types with neither party offending the other. In some cases, a minor tiff occurs and nothing more. In some cases, a battle for survival occurs.

Some microbes are too violent for our liking.

What determines variability in microbe virulence? In other words, what determines the relationship between man and the microbes? Why can't it be always nice—wouldn't that be a happier place to live? A lot of evolutionary philosophy underlies this phenomenon which we will address as we go along.

Microbes are not as weak as you think. They have a different face when it comes to hostility. Though unicellular, their punches carry a ton of weight. For example, one type of bacteria called Clostridium botulinum is a deadly pathogen. The science journal *Nature* carried an editorial recently that mentioned that botulinum is a killer and only 400 grams of this toxin are needed to kill off 7.8 billion humans. That is the size of a block of butter you buy in the supermarket.

I don't understand why mankind thinks we control the planet. Weight for weight, I do not think we have weapons or devices that can deliver botulinum's level of annihilation, not even nuclear. This tiny bacterium has something more deadly than our nukes.

Are microbes criminals in Nature's court?

The answer is a resounding No.

They are as keen to survive as any other lifeform on our planet. In exercising survival tactics, you cannot blame them for using the laws of Nature. Even in our own justice system an act of self-defense is not punishable (even if you kill). Microbes evolved various ways of deceiving our immune system to invade us and do the same for other life forms too. It is not true that microbes target only Homo sapiens.

All life systems are viewed as potential competitors by the microbes. They are also seen as a safe haven for their survival. Both are true. When we talk of invasion, microbes do not automatically cause disease or death—there are other outcomes too. It could be a harmless symbiosis. Or it could be mild trouble for a short period when the host suffers minor ailments.

The other extreme could be debilitating illness lasting for a prolonged period and finally even death.

Why is there such a variation in microbe's relations with other life systems? Why is it not uniform?

To me it looks like man and microbes do not lead lives of peace and tranquility. It is more like an international treaty (an inter-life treaty) with certain terms which should not be contravened.

No country conducts foreign affairs out of love for other countries. It is a tight-rope walking exercise that balances our interest with that of fellow countries. In the same way, man and microbes etched a plan based on how we relate to each other.

This plan is quite action-packed and there is never a moment of dullness.

Target life systems (hosts) are by no means sitting ducks. They evolved a diverse set of tactics to counter the offensive from microbes. This is legal in the court of law of Mother Nature.

What intrigues me is the reason why Corona virus would want to hurt us. It is not trying to rob us. It is not going to build an empire. Then why do they do this?

The rivalry between us and the microbes is not a new thing. They have always hated us. Homo sapiens have only been around for the past 200,000 years or so. Viruses and other microbes have existed for hundreds of millions of years.

In terms of evolutionary seniority, microbes are super senior to us. They have been around approximately 3 billion years and kind of feel *they* own the Earth. We are probably seen as newcomers trying to occupy their land. You see this when native populations of a land mass are disturbed by exploiters. This has happened in every part of the world and still happens.

Are the microbes ragging us because we intrude in their space? Is that why they cause diseases by infecting us? Do you know that every year 15-16 million people die all over the world from all kinds of microbial infections? Why this killing spree?

Microbial infections are considered medical problems. They are looked at as diseases that need medical treatment. This standard view is held by most of us. We try to prevent microbial infections by practicing hygiene—a concept we have known only for the past 150 years or so. Before that, man did not even know microbes existed—let alone their role in causing infections.

Man lived more like a wild animal until very recently. Even running water for bathing was unavailable in Europe until 18th century. I am told that Portugal was the first nation to have running water in Europe. Once I was a tourist visiting Lisbon and during a sight-seeing tour of Lisbon, the tour guide said that the Portuguese people bathed only three times in their lives— first at the time of birth, second on the day of marriage and the final one at the time of death. This might seem incredible, but this information shows that historically, mankind was never as hygienic as he is now.

I see microbial infection as a biological war between man and microbe. For that matter, man is not the only life form infected by microbes. All sorts of multicellular and unicellular life forms get infected by microbes. Whichever life form gets infected, the basis of that infection is the attempt made by the microbe to find an abode for survival. It is a land of honey and milk for these microbes to find a place to live inside man or some other well-to-do life form. There, the microbe will have a 24/7 supply of nutrients and a place to live at no cost.

What else could a microbe desire?

One imagines these microbes making the most of illegally occupying a man's body. When you are a houseguest, you are normally on your best behavior. You do not want your host to be inconvenienced. The situation is different when you pay to be a guest—then you have the right to expect comforts and provisions.

Staying in a hotel is a good example. You want comfort and good service from the hotel and the hotel expects you to benefit them by giving them money. This is a mutually beneficial relationship biologists call symbiosis. The truth is there are an awful lot of organisms living out there in perfect symbiotic relationships. There are many cases which organisms exploit other organisms—called parasitosis by which biologists—where the relation between the two organisms is unilaterally beneficial.

Why can't the man-microbe relationship be one of symbiosis rather than the antibiosis we see with pandemic viruses? To be honest, even parasitosis would be okay if the pandemic viruses didn't kill, but merely exploited.

This is what intrigues me the most.

Lethal intentions do not have any logic.

All is fair in love and war they say. Evolution endorses this view. For the sake of survival, the meanest tactics are allowed. No organism can be blamed for being predatory. It is biologically entitled to be predatory and there need be no qualms about the plight of the victim organism. Evolution comes to the aid of the victims too. Victim organisms are endowed with evasive tools and mechanisms, so they give a tough fight. If you look at the world, you see biological battles everywhere.

It is a gory place, this Earth.

Based on the argument above we cannot find fault with viruses like Corona for being so deadly (or at least perceived to be deadly). What do you do? Are you totally like Buddha or something preaching peace when Corona virus or some other microbe enters your fortress through illegitimate means (but perfectly legitimate means from the point of view of the intruding microbe as endorsed by evolutionary forces)? You unleash brutal force against the microbe through your immune system, your defense forces.

It is amazing that the tiny, invisible virus or bacteria never thought twice invading you who unashamedly possesses an army of billions of white blood cell soldiers. We all play the survival game by the biological rules. We are perfectly within biological laws when we are armed and dangerous. No one will arrest you for being in possession of deadly weapons. No criminal court of your state will put you behind bars for killing microbial victims—whereas you will be incarcerated for life for taking one human life.

Obviously, biological laws are different from social laws. You can kill any number of other life systems but never ever harm one of your own. The funny thing is when you want to kill masses of people at once it is perfectly allowed in the name of war. You could be celebrated as a hero and rewarded with bravery medals. The governments unashamedly find the required money for funding a war (even if borrowed) whereas getting a small research grant from it would be a Herculean task.

There you go.

My question is why, with your mighty army of billions of human beings, each with billions of white blood cell soldiers, did you cowardly take to your heels? We are afraid of fighting an invisible virus. We hid ourselves in our homes. That is even stranger because this Corona can kill only 2 or 3 out of every hundred it colonizes. It is not a seriously deadly pathogen.

Yet, our battle with Corona continues. Either we die or they die. Does biological war have to be always deadly? Isn't there room for moderation? Or, even better, is there room for tolerance towards one another?

Tolerance to microbes would be okay if they did not cause the inconvenience of disease and death. When the microbe causes unwanted pain and suffering, then how can we keep quiet? Even when I said the Corona virus is not deadly, I meant that 97-98% of people survive the infection. This is not because the Corona virus is merciful. It is only because our defense system i.e., our immunity, was powerful enough to beat them.

People with strong immunity can beat the virus and remain totally asymptomatic. A proportion of people with moderate immunity take a hit, show symptoms and might get ill enough to require hospitalization, but eventually they succeed in the battle. Only very weak people, especially with co-morbidities, are the ones who cannot survive the viral onslaught.

The Corona virus is said to cause lung infection (Pneumonia) like so many other microbes. It was alleged that causing lung inflammation was the primary mechanism by which Corona virus kills. But, as we learned more about the virus, it has been reported that the primary mechanism by which Corona virus kills may not be something the virus does. It is the massive attack launched by our bodies releasing and excess abundance of immune system mediators called Cytokines.

Cytokines are the effectors (or executors) of the immune system soldiers. They are molecular weapons hurled at the virus. Generally, any sort of infection or inflammation is met with some Cytokine release from the immune system as part of host defense. Cytokines are part of an elaborate, complicated, cascade initiated by the microbe-targeted immune action. The T lymphocytes are the ones that secrete these cytokines and there are quite a few of them.

Interferon Gamma is the primary cytokine that has anti-virus potential. There are a whole lot of others that can get activated and released when the complex network of immune system goes in full swing. It is true that our immune system often uses excessive force—probably incommensurate with the capacity of the enemy.

For each and everything, our immune system makes a fuss and overreacts. It may sound silly to lament about how our evolution-honed immune system overkills.

But it is true.

Otherwise, you would not see so many anti-inflammatory drugs like Brufen being used. Every time we have an injury, or twist our ankle, or have a swelling, we immediately take Brufen or another anti-inflammatory drug.

If you have surgery, your doctor will prescribe an anti-inflammatory drug to keep the surgical wound from swelling up and causing pain. In many cases, the doctors go for Steroid drugs which are a scale above the regular anti-inflammatory drugs.

Steroids basically suppressor our immune system. They are used as a standard regimen when treating inflammatory conditions—including autoimmune diseases. What the doctor is trying to do is to put the brakes on the run-away immune system. Otherwise, the collateral damage to our body due to excessive immune force would be far greater than the damage due to the disease itself.

In short, what I am trying to say is that it is no secret that our immune system is like a beast that needs to be tamed. By using anti-inflammatory drugs or immunosuppressive steroids, we try to paradoxically interfere with our own immune defense.

We do same-side goals when competing with a microbe or something noxious. How is that logical? My conclusion is that our immune system is like a roller-coaster ride that cannot be controlled in a fine manner or abruptly. Or it could be that this is the case with at least a significant proportion of people where too much brute force is unleashed more than required.

In the case of Corona virus infection, it was argued that this excessive Cytokine release (also called Cytokine storm) is the culprit that causes death of the patient—and not the lung damage caused by the virus itself. Can you believe that? And you want to blame the Corona virus?

Do we humans always behave so rudely towards all microbes? If we did so, the resources needed for microbial wars would be unimaginably high. The consequence of collateral damage will be too high to handle. By the grace of God we are not always so violent.

The Secret World of Microbes

There are many microbes living on and in different parts of our body all the time. They are called Normal Flora or Commensals. On our skin alone there are over 1,000 types of different bacteria living happily without causing any damage or disease to us.

Surprisingly, our ever-so-violent immune system turns a blind eye toward them. That is because these skin bacteria do some good to us. They create competition for harmful bacteria that want to colonize the skin for malicious reasons.

By creating this competition, the harmless skin bacteria drive out the harmful bacteria. Ultimately, this is purely a conflict between these 1,000 types of harmless skin bacteria and several other harmful bacteria for occupation of the skin land.

By winning this conflict, the harmless bacteria give us some benefit. They saved us from the hassle of dealing with the harmful bacteria which, given the propensity of the immune system to brute force, would have consumed useful resources that could have been spent elsewhere for constructive purposes.

What do the harmless bacteria get back? They get juicy, fatty, nutritious secretions from our skin. It is like the nectar that flowers offer to bees for spreading their pollen.

Our skin is the fortress of our body. It is our first line of defense against intruders. By keeping a watch on the skin fortress, these harmless bacteria do something very useful for us. Every now and then our skin wall is breached. This happens when we have a minor abrasion, or tear of the skin, due to an injury.

The gap in the skin fortress is an open invitation for the microbes. In many cases the microbes make a hurried entry. We try to prevent this by applying an antibiotic ointment or Iodine solution. Or we cover the broken skin with a plaster. If we are not careful the wound becomes infected, which means enemy microbial armies have successfully invaded our body.

When a wound is infected, it becomes purulent (pus)—an ugly sight. People look at pus in disgust. Little do we realize that the pus is dead white blood cells (hence the white, creamy color). These white cells which fought valiantly for you, to protect your skin fort, die away as unsung heroes.

The trouble with entry of microbes through the gaping holes in the skin is that it becomes relatively easier for them to hitch-hike a ride around the body through the blood sea. This situation is a state of emergency for the body. Medics call this Sepsis. It means potential multi-organ infections can ensue. It is potentially fatal, and doctors must treat Sepsis as quickly as possible—literally every hour counts.

Our gut is another place where we have lots and lots of harmless microbes living happily without causing discomfort or disease. We have similar harmless commensals in our mouth, windpipe and genitals as well. Because these parts of the body are exposed to the external environment, microbes find it easy to colonize.

Bacteria living in the gut (called gut flora) have gained immense attention in the last couple of decades. Literally, hundreds of research papers come out every year on the role of gut bacteria in health and disease. Apart from bacteria, even fungi and viruses live in our gut. Hundreds of microbial species are said to inhabit the human gut making it a very complex ecological niche.

Each of the microbial species may run into billions in population count making the total population of microbes living inside our gut outnumber the total number of human cells in our body. Our body is said to contain up to 30 trillion cells. Our gut is said to contain at least 25% more microbes than the 30 trillion and that is a huge number. A human being is really a super-organism not just made of our own type of human cells but a wide variety of microbes as well. We are a union of life systems.

One can call a human body the Union of Socialist Republic of Man and Microbes (USRMM).

Each human cell contains about 30,000 functioning genes. We must multiply this number by 30 trillion to get the total number of genes operating inside our body to carry out bodily tasks. Microbes, depending on their type, have anything from 10 to 1,000 genes inside them. If we multiply this number by the total number of microbes living inside the gut, then the total number of microbial gene programs will far outweigh human gene codes. Are we humans really hosts or is our relationship with gut microbes a different sort of arrangement?

The gut microbial community could be called Gut Microbiome—an entity on its own with a special status more than just commensal microbes. In fact, it is amazing how much is known about the gut micro-biome. It is said there is a connection between the gut microbial function and human mind called the Gut-Brain Axis. There are interactions between gut microbes and the central and enteric nervous system (intestinal nerve ganglions).

Autism, anxiety-depressive behaviors and functional gastrointestinal disorders are said to be the result of this gut-brain connection. Irritable bowel syndrome, a common intestinal ailment affecting so many worldwide, is a disorder linked to the gut microbes. It is said that even immunity is influenced by gut microbes and a lot of food allergies are a result.

The gut is a fertile place for life forms due to the nature of the food handling activity going on there. Food is there 24/7 and comes with no action required—what else could microbes ask for? Deep in the lower intestine there is little oxygen. Microbes that live there are anaerobic i.e., they live without oxygen. Human feces contain 100 billion bacteria per gram of stool.

About 30% of solid mass of feces is bacteria.

Given the abundance of bacteria and other microbes in the gut, it is reasonable to suspect they probably contribute to the cause of human life. Members of the gut micro-biome can synthesize Vitamin K and most of the water-soluble B complex vitamins such as cobalamin, folate, pyridoxine, riboflavin and thiamine. It is noteworthy that humans cannot make these vitamins by themselves, but we're very reliant on them for our metabolism.

Bacteria live in the gut and make themselves useful—which works fine for humanity. This is a fruitful and beneficial relationship between man and the microbe. Why can't pandemic viruses and bacteria play nice instead of being murderous?

It is down to the inter-species skills between organisms. Even when we deal with fellow humans, our affinity towards people is varied. Some people are easy to get along with, some are helpful, some are non-committal, some are annoying, and some are outright disgusting.

Life systems too have the same spectrum in their interactions with other life systems. They cannot be always nice to every other life system. They cannot always be helping them with deeds. They cannot always be tolerant.

One of the other contributions made by the microbes living in the human gut is the same as what the skin normal flora does. The harmless gut bacteria prevent harmful microbes from settling in the gut by fighting them off. As in the case of skin, it is a battle for occupying the gut land. The harmless bacteria fight the harmful bacteria for their benefit. They do not for a moment think about saving you. But a beneficial outcome of their selfish battle is that the harmful bacteria are unable to thrive in our gut and cause disease and suffering.

The gut is an open space. Gut microbes live there as if they were living in a gutter. Our immune system does not really work there—if at all. Consider the gut as an extension of the environment. By living there, microbes are not trespassing.

Only when microbes enter the gut lining wall do they become subject to immune hatred. Until then, the bacteria and other microbes are treated by our immune system as if they were not even part of your body. We just leave them alone. That is one unique relationship.

For that matter, even the skin-living microbes are treated as if they were part of the external environment because—technically speaking—the skin bacteria are outside the wall of your house. You shouldn't argue or fight someone standing outside your door. Skin bacteria are like dogs guarding your house.

It is common for countries to poke their noses into other country's politics or internal affairs—sometimes grooming and abetting terror groups to cause nuisance or even to destabilize a country's leadership. Much of the international terrorism going on in the world right now can be traced back to international interference and facilitation thanks to some nations. This sounds bad, but terrorism sometimes occurs inside our bodies.

One such instance is the dietary habit of eating yogurt. Do you view eating yogurt as warfare?

Let me explain.

Yogurt is a broth containing a good bacteria called Lactobacillus. It contains a few other types, but Lactobacillus is predominant. Yogurt is considered a probiotic—meaning it has content conducive to life. Basically, Lactobacillus and/or other bacteria produce lactic acid which then acts on the milk casein—curdling it.

This is why yogurt is also known as curd.

The bacteria in yogurt also make vitamins. So, a common dietary item in our daily life is the handiwork of bacteria. But that is not what I want to highlight when I mentioned we are facilitating bitter warfare in our own body like the countries do in international politics.

Lactobacillus and other harmless bacteria in yogurt produce Bacteriocins—substances that can kill a lot of harmful bacteria including the drug-resistant ones. By eating yogurt, we facilitate a bitter war between harmless and harmful bacteria.

When we eat yogurt, we send the gut an army of Lactobacillus. That army is expected to clobber the harmful bacteria causing a menace inside the gut. We then follow the same strategy that international leaders follow to further their goals.

It is said that yogurt is a good home remedy when someone has diarrhea. The reason is: it helps defeat the bacteria that upsets the intestine—leading to diarrhea. Normally, people have gastrointestinal upsets when they eat unhygienic food. That is because the food or drink they had at the restaurant may have been contaminated with some pathogenic, harmful bacteria.

Yogurt is an effective agent to control the growth of these harmful bacteria inside the gut. Eating yogurt is biological warfare at its best.

Each person's gut micro-biome is not the same. The

bacterial composition of the gut plays a major role in diseases like inflammatory bowel diseases, autism, anxiety-depression and food allergy. Some say body weight is controlled by gut bacteria.

The right combination of bacteria can make a person fat or slim. These sorts of experiments have been conducted in mice. Two gut bacteria are associated with lean body weight. Akkermansia muciniphilia and Christensenella minuta are linked to preventing weight gain. Akkermansia bacteria are boosted by foods such as cranberries, black tea, fish oil, bamboo shoots, flax seeds and rhubarb extract. The ratio of two other types of gut bacteria determines who will be fat and who will be slim.

Prevotella is a type of bacteria that digests fiber and carbohydrates. Bacteroidetes is another type of bacteria seen in people who eat more animal proteins and fat. If you have more Prevotella bacteria than Bacteridetes, then you are likely to be slim. Eating foods rich in fiber helps boost Prevotella bacteria.

It is said that exercise alters intestinal bacteria in humans and increases microbial diversity. Exercise increases the microbes that reduce inflammation, decreases insulin resistance and supports a healthy metabolism.

The intestinal microbiome is involved in the initiation and development of colorectal cancer. It's been proven that those profound modifications in the gut microbiome during the progression of colorectal cancer points to the role of bacteria in this cancer. Two types of bacteria, E. coli and Bacteroides fragilis, each contain a gene for producing a cancer-causing toxin known to be primary culprits.

Fusobacterium is another type of bacteria seen in a third of bowel cancers.

While talking of intestinal microbes it is worth mentioning the Cholera pandemics that rattled mankind many a times over the last many centuries. This is a good example of a bacterial pandemic as opposed to viral pandemics like Flu, Smallpox etc.

Our bodies and Cholera bacteria do not get along well. Cholera bacteria live in dirty water. When we consume unhygienic and unclean water, Cholera bacteria strikes. Often, unclean water is an indication of crowded and unsanitary living conditions. As always, microbes strike under such conditions. Perhaps this is a cybernetic feedback inhibition on the growth of human society to reduce population density. This is purely my theoretical conjecture, but it deserves some thought.

Between 1817 and 1824, Cholera pandemic struck Calcutta, India. It also spread also to South Asia, East Africa, Middle East and Mediterranean countries and killed 2-8 million people. The second wave of the Cholera pandemic came between 1826 and 1837 hitting America and Europe. The third wave came between 1846 and 1860 devastating Africa. So, over the last 200 years, Cholera bacteria invaded mankind 6 times claiming millions of lives.

In the last few years, it made a worrying appearance in Yemen. Looking back, Cholera was described in Indian chronicles even in the 5th century BC. Hippocrates described Cholera in Greece around the same time. Cholera was also described in the 15th century AD by the Portuguese in Bangladesh and India around the Ganges belt.

It is said that people died of diarrhea within a matter of hours. In short, Cholera is a microbe that hit mankind time and again for the last two millennia. People may not have known the exact cause of the diarrhea, but the symptoms described in the chronicles lead us to assume the disease indeed was Cholera.

Lactobacillus, the yogurt microbe, is a microbe. Cholera microbe is also a microbe. Both live in the human gut. One is a tame little creature and the other a serial killer.

Why this variation in man-microbe relation?

Is it the fault of the Cholera microbe that it chose to attack and kill rather than help us? Is it possible that if they chose a helpful attitude, we would be at peace? It does not look like we spare the cholera microbe—it is more likely the other way around. Cholera bacteria lets some people live while wiping out others.

We may overcome the Cholera bacteria with better sanitation methods. On the other hand, we farm lactobacillus and cultivate it in the form of yogurt. That creates a special relationship between us and Lactobacillus.

Wouldn't it be nice if other microbes lived so amicably with us?

The simple answer to the conundrum is that the microbe should avoid bad intentions when they deal with us. They should not irritate us by mischief. It should be gentle, mildly reactive and above all, lend a helping hand. Then we leave them alone and our immune system does not bother them. Only when the microbe is a criminal does the immune system make the relationship sour by initiating a deadly attack.

If the microbe was peace-loving then we would be peace-loving too.

This can be said of all pathogenic, harmful microbes. By killing their host, they put their free ride into jeopardy. When will they realize that? Or are they not supposed to realize that?

If life systems could live together peacefully, then there is enough for everyone to share on this planet. Man fought countless wars in the last 6,000 years. We have killed millions of our own kind. If that is the case, then how can we even raise the question about why the microbes kill us? Quite often when a greedy emperor invades a foreign land, he makes sure that he loots the occupied land and, often, destroys the people's lives by burning their houses down, destroying their culture etc.

A lion hunts down a deer for food. When the Corona virus or Cholera bacteria kill us, it is not for food. So, the nature's law that you are legally, morally and biologically allowed to kill other lifeforms for food is contravened.

This is like legitimization of killing for armed forces but not for civilians. If food is not the endpoint of the killer instinct of some microbes, then what is? They are surely not interested in wealth or land or power. This is where I am beaten.

Many people on our planet are vegetarians. They do not like to kill animals for food. Chicken, beef and lamb are products of animal kill. Vegetarians prefer to eat plants or drink renewable milk or eat renewable butter or cheese that can be obtained from the milk. This approach is different from slaughtering the cow and eating it as beef.

My intention is not to judge who is morally right. It is common sense to keep your provider alive. This common sense went amiss in the case of microbes. I suppose they are not supposed to think. I also suppose that on that basis, terrorists make the same mistake as killer microbes by causing death and destruction to their own people and country.

Some microbes are totally harmless. Some cause minor disturbances to our health and then go away. Regular Flu virus is one such. It is amazing that the Flu virus is a distant cousin of this Corona guy. How different are they? Don't you find two brothers having diametrically opposite characters?

Some microbes cause a prolonged infection without killing. Some are outright killers. Microbes use our body as their playground for all sorts of games.

It is possible that we attack the microbes too hard once they enter our body. Brute force may cause these microbes to evolve defense strategies that include murder. If we did not use so much brutal immune force, maybe microbes would tone down their defense.

It is well-known that many of our immune responses are so overboard that there is a lot of collateral damage to our cells. That is why doctors prescribe anti-inflammatory drugs to subside swelling and pain caused by fiery immune attacks.

Our anti-microbial defenses are twin-edged weapons capable of causing self-damage. We need to evolutionarily learn how to control our aggression toward microbes.

I suspect over a period (possibly millions of years) most microbes would have learnt to co-live with man rather than kill.

I can't help but think of terrorist movements as unavoidable manifestations of yet-to-be-perfected tolerance between ideological groups in the human society. Terrorist groups could be viewed purely as aggressive pushers of their ideology.

As a random example, let's look at Maoism. When someone is classified as a Maoist, it simply means they belong to a group that are overzealous followers of Mao Tse Tung, the Chinese Communist revolutionary, who became the founding father of the Republic of China.

Unfortunately, Maoists are viewed as terrorists by political establishments. I feel this is the same misunderstanding seen between microbes and man. We view microbes as things to be terminated. Our immune system is designed and geared towards this goal. This view does not change until the microbe demonstrates its allegiance to a holy relationship with man by virtue of a beneficial contribution. Then the human immune system moderates its outlook on this particular microbe. Maybe we have not lived together long enough for such tolerance to develop. In Mao Tse Tung's China, the capitalists were the terrorists. They were fought against. Now, tolerance toward capitalistic terrorism is accepted as normal in China.

One of the other curious aspects of man-microbe relations is opportunism. Microbes colonizing the human body, referred to as commensals or normal flora, behave differently when the human body is weak. They are well-behaved and obedient as long as our body is strong and our immune system is intact.

But some people end up with a weakened immune system due to the exhaustion of frequent infections and the toll it takes on the immune soldiers. Sometimes, even excessive intake of immunosuppressive medications like steroids weakens the immune system making us vulnerable to attack from pathogens.

AIDS microbes deliberately hit our CD4 and CD8 cells—weakening our immune system. In such immunosuppressed individuals, the so-called normal flora microbes show their different face.

They attack us when they know we are too weak to fight back. This raises a question. Was there real affinity between man and the so-called harmless microbe or is it a case of deception and cunning?

For this same reason, terrorism and internal strife are rampant in economically and politically debilitated countries. Terror groups and political dissidents keep quiet in a country that is strong. Many African nations would fit the description of people with a weakened immune system.

We live in a world where relationships between entities will always be imperfect. We will be forever learning how to be amicable with all around us. This is the new normal paradigm that has been mooted to handle the Corona virus.

Imagine how much change has happened since Corona came. We wore masks in public places. We were unable to sit and have a relaxed drink in a bar or a Cafe. We could not go out for a nice dinner. We could not go to the theatre.

The list goes on. They say that this is the new normal.

This is like living in the middle of terror groups who made a new normal in several ways. For instance, we face rigorous security checks at the airport. They ask us to empty our pockets, remove our shoes, throw away our water and other liquids, scan our luggage and so on.

Above all this, they check our passports and insist on photo identity documents. As recently as the 1980s, air travel was not like this. What we see now is the new normal of air travel which we silently accept.

Even the use of computers is not the same. Computers are not so old. We've had this technology for only about 50 years. We are always wary of using a computer in public places because social distancing is impossible between your computer and another guy's computer.

Your WIFI could be picked up by some random guy sitting near you. You could be exposed to a hacker in your hotel room who sneaks into your computer through WiFi or some other virus or worm.

This is the same fear we have about a random person giving you the Corona virus by sitting nearby. Though we never called it that, the past 25 years have been all about creating new normals.

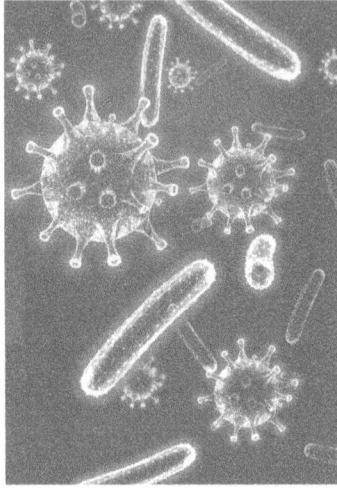

Chapter 4

MICROBIAL COLONIES ARE LIKE FEDERAL UNIONS OF STATES

IT APPEARS TO be a choice by Microbes to remain unicellular. Earlier, I asked why microbes remain single-celled while their descendants went on to become multi-cellular and more powerful. The argument that multi-cellular life forms are more prosperous and powerful is questionable. I alluded to this when I pointed out that single-celled life forms are more plentiful in numbers and mass.

I also suggested that some microbes have extraordinary abilities—such as eating atomic radiation. Above all, Nature requires execution of some tasks (such as fixing of atmospheric Nitrogen) that only unicellular life forms can do. You cannot have everyone become millionaires and bosses because we need someone to do the work.

Microbial unicellular systems exist in federal structures too. This is like the United States of America, the former USSR (Union of Soviet Socialist Republic), the European Union,

NATO (North Atlantic Treaty Organization), and the United Nations etc.

Unions of states in these federal structures are more for cooperation and partnership than governance. Microbes are known to live in such unions too—called a Biofilm. Biofilms are aggregations of millions of bacteria living as one entity. It looks like a multi-cellular life form but not quite. In a multi-cellular life form, the union of all the cells is mandatory and they are governed strictly by anatomical and physiological laws. A Biofilm is more of an optional arrangement beneficial to all participants. The dental plaque most of us have is a Biofilm—a bacterial colony living on your teeth. The bad breath we suffer from is the metabolic product of this bacterial colony eating your food. The bluish-green layer you see in wet bathrooms is also a bacterial Biofilm.

Bacterial colonies also form on other surfaces. When they grow on equipment used in medical practice it is a cause for concern because it is very difficult to get rid of them and pose a big risk for patients.

Bacteria living in a Biofilm colony have advantages. Defense is one of them. Individual bacteria need to do less to defend themselves. Defense becomes a federal responsibility. Individual bacteria can get rid of their individual cell walls used as a means of defense. This makes them less susceptible to antibiotics because most antibiotics work by hitting the cell walls of the bacteria.

This is a primary reason why Biofilms are tough to get rid of. It might take a 100-fold more antibiotic dose than normal to even tickle a biofilm—which, due to side-effects, is impractical.

It is said that more than 80% of human bacterial infections are caused by bacteria living in a biofilm which makes them difficult to treat. The usual antibiotics may work initially, but the bacteria rebound. Wounds are difficult to treat for the same reason: because 90% of chronic wounds and 6% new wounds have some sort of Biofilms.

Bacterial colonies inside a biofilm are closely monitored for controlling the population as well as for adjusting the density of bacteria. There are internal conduits inside the colony like roads for the distribution of resources. Many times, bacterial colonies are populated by other microbial species which gives them a cosmopolitan character. The needs of bacterial cells in a colony, external threats, and density of bacteria are all monitored using molecular sensors. One can compare this to a city council that plans welfare measures based on the needs of the residents and the locality. City councils often conduct public surveys, more like opinion polls, to gather vital information for the purpose of making informed plans for social welfare. A city council will hardly listen to an individual petition. As an example, for action to take place, there must be a reasonable number of people who petition for a service improvement.

This majority opinion carries more weight than an individual opinion. Molecular sensing of bacterial colony needs is called Quorum Sensing by microbiologists. This helps the colonies divide their tasks amongst members.

For instance, metabolic programs can be divided, and no individual bacteria need rely entirely on their own genes. Bacteria living in a Biofilm can afford to run only some of their programs and can get others to supply them with products of programs they did not run.

This is cooperation.

Which genes will be active, and which will be shut off is determined by Quorum Sensing.

One gram of dental plaque can contain as many as 100 billion bacterial cells. This is a bigger number than the total number of Homo sapiens who ever lived on the planet Earth! It is mind-boggling! And keep in mind that these bacteria usually replicate every 20 minutes!

It is said that 98% of all bacteria live in Biofilms which indicates that bacteria do not live like single-celled organisms at all. They deceive us. Instead, they prefer to live in a loose, federal union of bacteria. It is said that more than half the biomass on the planet Earth lives in biofilms.

That says something, doesn't it?

This answers a question I raised a little while ago. Single-celled organisms chose to remain unicellular but at the same time they enjoy the benefits of cellular unions not much different from multicellular life forms.

Single-celled organisms find advantages in this arrangement, otherwise evolution would not have selected it.

It appears that viruses enjoy a social relationship with fellow viruses. Reminiscent of multicellular life, they communicate with each other. When they attack an enemy (host), the viral soldiers chat with each other about the events at the battlefront. They use their own molecular language for this purpose. This is like coded communications that soldiers use to transmit secret messages on the battlefield.

Scientists who study viral communication methods coined the term Arbitrium to describe this. Arbitrium is a six-amino-acid-long viral protein. It is believed the viral soldiers use species-specific code languages. We recognize about 15 viral code languages. Primarily, these coded communications between viruses determine when to attack and when to go dormant.

Imagine a virus attacking a bacterial target. Each virus announces that it hit a target. After replication, the virus breaks open the bacterial walls and releases its offspring. These offspring attack further bacterial targets and so on.

There comes a point when there are no new bacterial targets left—at that time, the viruses send out messages to slow down.

This message is interpreted by viruses to stay dormant in their last target—as if in hiding. This is like the lockdowns we experienced during the COVID-19 pandemic—where people stayed in, or close to, their homes.

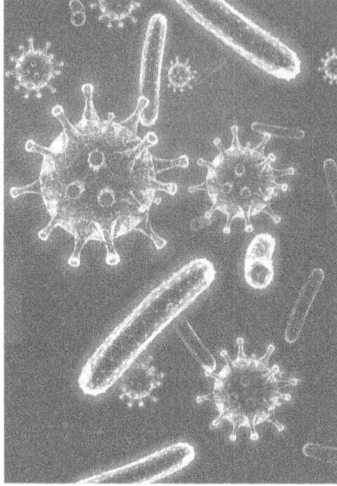

Chapter 5

HIDE AND SEEK: HOW MICROBES AND HOSTS MUTUALLY EVADE EACH OTHER

SOME VIRUSES RESIDE benignly inside human cells for long periods. The Hepatitis virus is one such. It causes inflammation of the liver leading to jaundice. These Hepatitis viruses can remain inside the liver cell even for decades. Long residency is not good for the human host because it contributes to liver cancer.

The Polio virus is another example. It can exist in the human host for years by hiding in human nerve cells.

Also, the Herpes virus can permeate nerve cells for long periods.

Bacteria can also take long-term residency in human victims. TB bacteria can do it for years. Another bacterium belonging to the same family is the one that causes Leprosy. This bacterium also is a squatter.

These squatter bacteria and viruses spend years inside our

cells without paying any rent whatsoever. I used the word rent as a symbol of something given back in return. In most cases of symbiotic relationships, the squatters pay back in kind. They do something of value to the host in return for using their resources. But TB bacterium gives us nothing but trouble by slowly eating away the lungs. TB bacterium has affected man since time immemorial. It has been a killer for centuries. It is said that nearly a third of the world population is latently infected with the TB bacteria—that is one out of every three people on the planet.

TB bacterium has a trick up its sleeve to squat undisturbed. They defy our defense forces inside the body. Macrophages are one type of cell in our body. Their job is defense. They are part of our innate immune system helping us to attack invading microbes. They have the characteristic ability to engulf the unwanted microbe and deliver them to a chamber inside the cell called Lysosomes. Lysosomes are the equivalent of cellular hell. They are like the dungeons in medieval time prisons where the prisoners were tortured in a variety of cruel ways.

Lysosomes roast the microbe under extremely acidic/oxidative conditions and melt it down. This is like what our religions say about the judgment day when you will be thrown into boiling oil in hell. It is judgment day for microbes. TB bacteria learned a trick or two over time about how to tackle this human defense menace. It hacks into the cellular Lysosome cauldron programs and inactivates it. The macrophages then become toothless snakes. TB bacteria reside happily for ever after inside them. Just imagine a medieval prisoner sitting right inside the dungeon and enjoying the stay.

As a defense against microbes, plants also make inhibitors of microbial toxin called efflux pumps. One could imagine the efflux pump as a sort of mechanical device. These efflux pumps are made of molecules. It is basically nanotechnology. Microbes have an incredible ability to dodge the antibacterial substances we use against them. What they do, which you might find very difficult to believe, is use their efflux pumps to expel the anti-bacterial substances that enter their body.

These efflux pumps are evolutionarily conserved across many life forms. They are on the list of survival tools that are essential for life systems. It is like a household having certain essential items like umbrella, candle or torch light, an alarm system etc.

The purpose of this molecular pump serves the biological need for expelling toxic substances. It is like using buckets to expel flood water that entered our houses. Lower organisms have these molecular efflux pumps to pump out toxic compounds entering their cells. This is an evolutionarily conserved technology. It is basically a defense mechanism.

Life systems are constantly exposed to many types of toxic substances in water, food and air. In our daily lives, humans are also exposed to many toxins. These include pollutants, chemicals and additives used in food and cosmetics, effluents from factories, medicines etc.

Handling and processing these unwanted toxic substances is called Xenobiotic metabolism. We humans have an elaborate detoxification system comprised of liver and kidneys that help us metabolize and excrete toxic compounds. Some life forms do not have this luxury. This is especially the case for microbes which have only one cell at their disposal. They do this job in different ways.

One way is the efflux pump that literally grabs the antibacterial substance hurled at them and pumps it out. Even cancer cells have this kind of efflux pump (a type of molecule called P-glycoprotein stationed on the surface of the cell) that throws out the cancer medicines. By doing so they become resistant to the drugs. But this is not the only mechanism by which microbes or cancer cells develop resistance to drugs.

In defense there is an attack and there is also a counterattack. This is universal. Plants found ways to counterattack the efflux pump strategy of microbes. They make inhibitors of these efflux pumps. By inhibiting the efflux pumps they make it difficult for the microbes to dodge the antibacterial defenses.

Plants make them and station them on top of their cell

walls. Pharmacological researchers are looking to exploit this plant technology for human medical use. It is possible that such inhibitors of microbial efflux pumps could be next-generation antibiotics.

As we see in nature, the tug-of-war between the prey and predator can lead to ingenious evasion strategies for both parties. If the plant, man or another life system scans the microbe for danger signals, they are looking for characteristic, tell-tale marks of the microbe called antigens.

Frequently, offensive actions are directed against these antigens only. These are like identification marks that we use to pinpoint a person's identity. The microbes use novel ways to conceal themselves to escape detection and shield their attacks.

One such evasive technique is the sequestration of antigens. This means they will tuck in their surface antigens to become invisible to the radar of the host life system. Or the microbes change the nature or appearance of the antigens by deliberately mutating them. This makes it confusing for the immune system to first identify the microbe and even if it was detected, the attack becomes ineffective because of the change in the antigenic structure. If a criminal changes hair color, clothing or haircut, it's harder for the police to catch them. Criminals even change their passport to escape detection.

Similarly, microbes can use an antigenic structure on the outside of their cells that mimic a host molecule. This is the ultimate disguise. Our cells have various surface receptors for allowing the entry of essential self-molecules. These are like ports of entry. They are guarded heavily. But microbes give the slip by mimicking a human molecule. They are that clever. When your immune cells look for microbial patterns, these humanoid molecule-bearing microbes are missed and are allowed in by the cell surface receptor ports.

The strategy of microbes to disguise themselves to look like a normal part of us is the same strategy used by hackers to send Trojans horses with concealed soldiers. They send an email or a message that seems genuine and you allow your computer to receive it and open it. Once you do that you are done. The same fate awaits the cell whose receptors open their gates thinking a delivery arrived from a legitimate source.

The basis of human-like molecules in microbial programs is bewildering. Why would a microbe have a molecule like ours when they cannot use it for its legitimate function?

For example, the Corona virus seems to have an ACE2-like molecule that allows it to dock onto the receptor for ACE2 in lung cells. The Corona virus must have acquired it some time ago when it historically interacted with human cells in some form or other. Corona viruses do not integrate with human DNA like retroviruses, so we cannot postulate that it acquired this extra bit of gene code during such an integration event. But one cannot dismiss the fact that it may have acquired this piece of gene code for making ACE2-like molecule from another virus of a different family.

I said earlier that microbes have the extraordinary capability to upload gene codes from other microbes or even from dead, free-floating DNA strands.

Streptococci bacteria can cause heart and kidney damage—sometimes years after the initial infection. This bacterium affects us by causing a sore throat. What is the relation between a throat infection bacteria and heart/kidney damage? This is because the streptococcus bacteria have a surface antigen called the M protein which is structurally like proteins in specific human tissues such as muscle (myosin), heart and kidney.

When our immune system initiates an attack against the streptococcus bacteria, our antibody weapons also hit our own tissues because they are similar to the streptococcal protein. That is why the affected patient can get heart and kidney damage.

Klebsiella and Shigella bacteria have molecules very similar to the HLA B27 molecule in our immune system. When we fight against these bacteria, antibodies we make can hit our own self-molecule. Patients can get joint damage because of the crossfire.

There are many examples of infectious diseases due to microbial entry into host cells through receptor uptake/internalization pathways meant for host molecules because of structural similarities. Various organisms have virulence factors/attachment factors that potentiate host cell entry due to sharing of structural similarities which enable use of host cell signal recognition machinery to gain entry.

For example, Staphylococcus aureus, a bacterium which is known to cause pyogenic skin infections, has receptors for binding host skin connective tissue molecules like fibronectin, laminin, and collagen because it has a structural adaptation.

Upon entering the skin's connective tissue, the bacteria settle and cause pus-producing skin boils.

Mycobacterium leprae, the causative bacterial agent for leprosy, binds host cell fibronectin—potentiating entry into nerve cells called the Schwann cells and epithelial cells. The lock-key relation holds here as in previous examples. Once settled, they start the protracted disease process that goes on for years.

Sometimes microbes use counter-offensive missiles to neutralize the antibodies. They secrete antigenic surface components into the soluble medium like decoys. What do our antibody bullets do? They shoot at these decoys. The bullets are wasted, and the bacterium carries on happily.

Do you believe me?

Streptococcus pneumoniae and Neisseria meningitides bacteria release capsular polysaccharides (sugars) as decoys to escape the fury of the antibodies. Some bacteria, like some species of Neisseria, Streptococcus and Hemophilus, produce enzymes that can break down and degrade our antibodies.

It is like anti-ballistic warfare. Staphylococcus bacterium can produce a substance that clumps IgG antibodies—inactivating them.

I can cite more examples of such microbial unraveling of host molecular structures with the intention of unlawful entry. If I did, this chapter would look like a discourse in microbiology and so I will stop.

Common herbs like Tarragon and Thyme contain Caffeic acid which is effective against viruses, bacteria and fungi. Plants are rich in a wide variety of products like tannins, terpenoids, alkaloids and flavonoids—all with antimicrobial properties. Use of medicinal plants for curing infections is age-old wisdom handed down across civilizations for centuries.

This is called Ethnopharmacology. Ancient people, and in many contemporary societies even today, use plant extracts to cure various ailments. Plants generally are the source of 25-50% of currently used modern pharmaceuticals, but none of them are used for antimicrobial purposes.

This is weird because there are many useful household remedies for warding off infections, including turmeric, garlic, pepper, Neem and ginger. They are tried and tested. Strangely, none of their active ingredients found their way into modern pharmacopoeia. But this situation might change in the near future as mainstream modern Medicine is increasingly receptive to plant-derived antimicrobials because currently used antibiotics are fast losing their steam.

Plants seem to have an endless ability to make aromatic molecules—mostly phenols or their phenol derivatives. Plants use them for defense against microbes, insects and herbivores.

The action of plant chemicals on microbes is of interest to us now, so I will not go into any depth about products made by plants to ward off insects and other animals that try to eat them.

Two examples of antimicrobial phenolic compounds are Catechol and Pyrogallol which have action against microorganisms.

Catechin is one such plant-derived antimicrobial substance. It is present in Oolong green teas. It is observed that teas have antimicrobial effect due to the mixture of catechin compounds in them. Catechins can even hit Cholera bacteria, one of the deadliest known microbes. Catechins can also fight other microbes like Shigella, which is another deadly intestinal bacterium.

Flavonoid compounds made by plants have inhibitory effects on multiple types of viruses. Whether they have been tested against Corona virus I do not know. We normally consume about 1 gram of flavonoids in our diet.

I cannot mention or describe each plant-derived chemical with medicinal value. My wish is to inform you that there are several organic chemicals made by plants that can beat microbes.

For plants, such antibacterial mechanisms constitute their immune system. After all, they too are susceptible to microbial attacks. We benefit from these plant-derived antibacterial products by consuming them as food. Ginger, garlic, turmeric, pepper, Basil leaves, etc. are common foodstuffs.

These plants give us the benefit of antimicrobial protection while at the same time serving a nutritional purpose. Sometimes I wonder whether these plants make these medicinal products only for their use or they are also intended for use by other life forms like us.

After all, don't plants give us all the food we need? Maybe they play a dual role—designed to give us nourishing food, but also medical protection.

This is not a far-fetched idea at all.

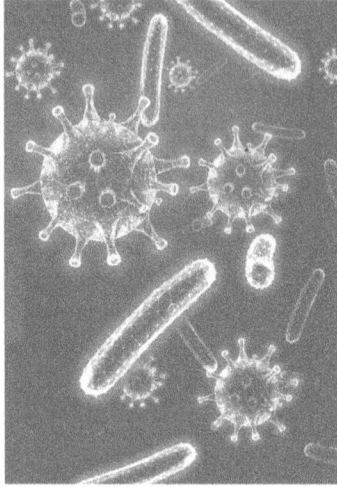

Chapter 6

CODE BREAKING: EAVESDROPPING ON MICROBIAL COMMUNICATIONS

A COUNTER-INTELLIGENCE MEASURE taken by governments against terrorists is surveillance of their communications. This enables government agencies to know what and where the next attack might be. By tapping emails, phones and coded messages passed along by other means, we monitor information exchanged between terrorists. We cannot do the same for microbial attacks because we do not understand the language of the microbes.

Microbes talk to each other—communicating a lot of information about what is going on at the battlefront, i.e., the host body. Microbes (both bacteria and viruses) have communication strategies that help them exchange vital information during an invasion. This helps them efficiently execute their attack.

If their covert communications are interrupted, the

microbes are unable to mount an effective attack. If only we knew their language, we could tap into their communication channels and take countermeasures. But there are other life systems—like plants—that can listen to microbial information exchanges.

Nature allows eavesdropping on microbial attacks by the victims of microbial attacks. Intelligence agencies in our modern society work by eavesdropping on criminals and terrorists. But, inside our body, we are unable to interrupt microbial communications because we have no means of decoding them. Surprisingly, other lifeforms have mastered the art of covert surveillance of microbial communication. Plants are one such lifeform. Plants are susceptible to such microbial infections and evolved strategies for defense.

As will be seen in detail later, we humans evolved an elaborate immune system to fight microbes. But, what about plants? How do they protect themselves? They subvert malicious microbes by listening to their plans.

Plants have several defense mechanisms. I want to talk about one such strategy that makes CIA and FBI strategies pale in comparison. It is said that plants can interfere with microbial communication and scramble the messages. This is like our war time tactics where we intercept enemy messages (which are coded), decipher them, and take actions accordingly to thwart an enemy attack. In some cases, we inactivate communication channels by destroying command centers so secret messages cannot be sent. It is not uncommon for counterintelligence to plant misguiding messages so enemy forces are confused and disoriented. When it comes to love and war, all is fair.

Researchers identified molecular message-scramblers used by plants. They use these molecular devices to scramble the messages sent as part of Quorum Sensing used in bacterial colonies. Quorum Sensing helps bacteria living in colonies exchange vital information to help them thrive. By inhibiting Quorum Sensing, plants thwart efforts to set up microbial strongholds. This finding has tremendous importance for us. Pharmaceutical companies find these plant-derived inhibitors of bacterial Quorum Sensing for potential next generation antibiotics—they could be seen in your pharmacies one day.

Plants are experts in deciphering communication codes used inside living networks like biofilms. This is because they are also capable of living in such networks. We humans also live in human networks called societies, but our communication methods are different between people.

We use languages which are phonetic skills totally different from the communication tools used by biofilms. That is why we do not know what bacterial biofilms talk about. Our other methods of communication—like emails, letters and SMS messages—would not work either, would they? You can't possibly use these tools to communicate with microbes.

We need to spend a little time trying to understand the extraordinary capacity of plants to do microbial surveillance. They evolved these strategies over time. Ignore purists who rebuke any attempt by people to talk of the ability of life systems as if it was a plan towards a goal. Purists feel this applies only to human species or those life forms that have a brain. All other life systems—without the brain—supposedly evolved certain characteristics by evolution happening only by random chance.

It does not matter if evolutionary mechanisms are perfectly tailor-made to solve survival problems. You are not allowed to think that goal-oriented planning took place. To be honest, I do not care about purists. I would only worry about them if I was writing a paper for a peer-reviewed journal. This book is not a peer-reviewed journal. It gives liberty to the human mind to wander in any direction the mind takes us. That is where the real excitement is.

Generally, trees have a longer life span than we do. It is common to see trees living for hundreds of years. A pine tree in California, US, is approximately 4,900 years old. To think they are of the same age as recorded human civilization is mind-boggling. This plant lived through the Egyptian, Greek, Minoan and Persian civilizations and still going strong.

Pine trees in Mount Read, Tasmania, apparently live in networks like bacterial biofilms. It is a tree colony made of clones. Thousands of trees grow and survive using the same root sources. This tree biofilm spans an area of 2.5 acres and is said to be about 10,000 years old.

A similar tree colony exists in the National Forest of Utah where a colony of trees spans as much as 105 acres. There are about 47,000 trees using the same root network underground. The roots of the trees are intertwined and are not separate for each tree. This tree colony is around 80,000 years old.

That is one hell of a length of time.

Mentioning examples of such tree networks is to show that the trees have the capability to communicate. Even when not living in such biofilms, trees are known to use chemical signals to communicate. That is why they understand the chemical languages of the bacterial biofilms. Black Walnut trees use a toxic chemical signal called Juglone to kill trees of the same kind trying to grow too near to them. This reduces the density of trees growing in a region and thereby helps avoid competition.

Some plants use air-borne chemicals to inform trees growing nearby that their branches are impeding sunlight, and they are not getting enough.

Sagebrush plants release camphor molecules in the air to inform other fellow trees that insects are attacking.

Plants communicate with microbes when they are engaged in symbiotic relationships. Fungi are generally known to grow on the roots of trees. When pests attack the trees, the affected plants communicate this information to other trees through the underground root-fungus network. No wonder trees know how to decipher microbial communication.

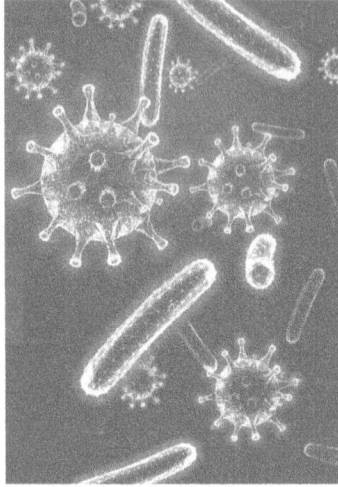

Chapter 7

GOOD MICROBES: MODERN ANTIBIOTICS ARE BASED ON TECHNOLOGY BORROWED FROM MICROBES

ANTIBIOTICS USED IN our hospitals were not invented by humanity. We discovered them by studying the environment. Who created them? That's an interesting question.

Antibiotics are a medical intervention technique that kills infection-causing microbes. But antibiotics have a totally unsuspected origin. They are molecular weapons made by some types of microbes to kill competing microbes. This is tribal warfare amongst microbes—a conflict between the microbes themselves. We exploit this microbial rivalry for medical purposes.

Microbes have existed for 3 billion years. In our current form, we have existed for just 200,000 years. Medical science is only about 200 years old. As I said, we did not invent antibiotics.

We didn't do painstaking research to create modern antibiotics. Well, in one sense we did—we painstakingly searched the environment for them. But, in another sense we took what was already out there in nature.

How could antibiotics exist in nature? Who made them? Why were they made?

Antibiotics are molecular weapons made by microbes to attack competing organisms that inhabit their ecosystem. These molecular weapons were made for combat purposes. Conflict between life systems is not new—it has been around for billions of years. We use guns, knives and bombs to ward off our enemies. Some life forms use poisons to kill their rivals.

Unicellular life forms like fungi evolved toxic substances to kill bacteria living in their territory. This was an evolutionarily gained skill. It is amazing that antibacterial substances are so intricately designed that stump organic chemists of world class universities.

Again, purists balk at the thought of purposeful design by fungi. They would feel more at ease if I just said the fungi arrived at the complex organic chemistry of antibiotic molecules by chance. It beats me why multinational pharmaceutical companies—investing billions of dollars and employing dozens of PhDs—cannot invent such crafty molecules. I worked in Pharmaceutical Research and Development for many years. I worked for a top 5 pharmaceutical company in the world. I know for a fact the so-called Lead Compounds used for developing new pharmaceuticals are almost always molecules purified from a natural source such as soil bacteria or plants. This applies to all sorts of diseases and not necessarily infectious diseases. This is an undeniable fact.

In the 1930s, Alexander Fleming accidentally discovered that a substance secreted by the fungus Penicillium killed the bacteria he was growing in a Petri dish in his lab. As it happened, Fleming had kept some bread somewhere near to the place he had his bacterial broth. That bread got stale and grew fungus on top—something we encounter regularly in our daily lives. This fungus forms a bluish green layer on top of the bread.

It happened that this fungal growth spread to the container containing the bacterial growth. Wherever this fungus settled on the Petri dish there was an inhibition of growth of the bacteria making Fleming suspect the fungus was making a substance that was fatal to the bacteria.

Later, other researchers purified the killer molecule from this fungus and named it as Penicillin. This Nobel Prize-winning discovery literally transformed the way we treat infections. Until then, people were died of simple infections. With the advent of Penicillin, it was possible to treat many infections and lives were easily saved.

As the years went by, researchers regularly screened soil samples for any microbes that might contain useful antibacterial or other medicinally active substances. This practice is still in vogue. Pharmaceutical companies collect soil and water samples from different parts of the world to isolate microbes and study them for presence of potential medicines.

Penicillin discovery was followed by the discovery of Streptomycin, the drug used for Tuberculosis. This antibiotic was identified in the microbial species called Streptomyces. The discovery of other antibiotics followed over the years.

Pharmaceutical companies created newer, semi-synthetic antibiotics by tinkering with the natural antibacterial substances and creating newer ones with additional properties.

One thought that comes to mind is pharmaceutical companies exploited the intellectual property of the microbes without paying any compensation. As a species, we benefited from this exploitation. We made our pharmaceutical formulary look respectable thanks to the microbes. Imagine a pharmaceutical company stealing the idea of a new medicine from a competitor. The victim will raise hue and cry and seek millions of dollars (possibly billions) in compensation from the unauthorized user. It is good that such things didn't happen when we plagiarized microbial pharmacology. It was freely available for everyone to use. It is God's gift to us.

It would not be an exaggeration to say that our modern medicine is a direct product of nature. 90% of all medicines we use for all kinds of diseases are derivatives of plants or other life forms. We use molecular technology perfected by other life forms for either self-defense or even benevolence (like using plants for food).

Maybe there is a medicine derived from natural sources for the Corona virus, but we have not identified it yet. There are many plant substances known to have antiviral properties, but none of them have been properly subjected to research to a level acceptable for approval by drug regulatory agencies.

This is partly because the bars are raised high by drug regulators. Citing patient safety, drug regulators forced pharmaceutical companies to conduct too many clinical trials—which make it very expensive to bring new medicines to the market.

We might have shot ourselves in the foot with overzealous caution for so-called safety. It was easier to find and bring out new medicines for human use until the 1970s and probably 1980s, but after that, too many hurdles hamper the process of bringing potentially new medicines to the pharmacy.

From an evolutionary perspective, antibiotics represent the struggle for life. They were made for self-protection by some microbes. This happened hundreds and possibly thousands of years ago when man did not exist—way before our species came about.

It is intriguing that antibiotics appear in our battle arsenal—helping us in our fight against microbes. Under the guise of modern medicine, we take credit for medical advances without acknowledging that we use products as old as the Earth—for which we have no right of claim of ownership.

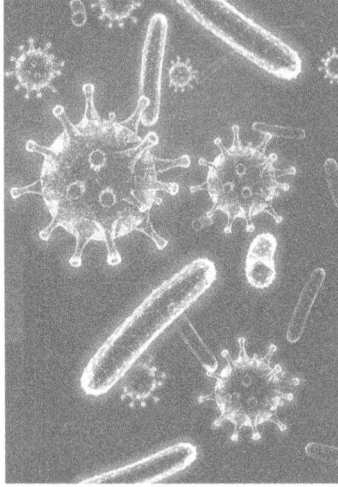

Chapter 8

STAR WARS: SHOOTING DOWN ANTIBIOTICS

WHEN AN INVADING lifeform makes a toxic product, it is logically expected per evolutionary principles, that the victim lifeform should find a way to defend itself. This is how nature works. No lifeform wants to be an easy victim for its enemies. The prey-predator relationship is one element of the constant battle for survival.

A substantial part of the survival game is preemptively striking against an enemy where the purpose is not food. The purpose is intentional annihilation of the enemy so the natural resources in the ecosystem are available for exclusive use of the attacker.

When attacked, life systems retaliate in self-defense. Where there is poison there will be an antidote. Some lifeforms even evolved protection against snake poison. This example illustrates the concept that, in the battle of life, defense is as important as offense. If microbes make antibiotics, then there surely should be retaliation from the target organisms the antibiotics were meant to kill.

Figuratively, this is similar to wearing a bullet-proof vest as protection against a bullet. Ronald Reagan, when he was US president, came up with the idea of Star Wars where he envisioned that a missile attack against US could be stopped by counter-offensive anti-ballistic missiles providing an impenetrable space shield.

This defense mechanism was necessitated by the technology wherein enemy nations, sitting far away, had the capability to strike with missiles with ranges of thousands of kilometers.

Naturally, countries developed anti-ballistic missiles to intercept and destroy these remotely delivered incendiary projectiles.

Conceptually, anti-ballistic missile technology is like a mosquito net or repellant creams that keep mosquitoes at bay. These strategies act as shields. I used the example of a mosquito—likening it to a missile. When a mosquito bites, you only lose a drop of blood, but do not discount the threat of biological warfare the tiny mosquito creates by carrying microbes in its blood—such as Malaria and other diseases. Mosquitos can be lethal. They can transmit several infectious microbes.

One point worth mentioning is that mosquitoes use heat detection for targeting and locating their targets. This same technology is used in defensive missiles. So, my comparison is not bad at all.

Microbes evolved molecules that can target and destroy the antibiotics hurled at them by enemy microbes. This is a natural phenomenon. To counterattack is their evolutionary right. I use the example of such anti-antibiotic missile warfare. Penicillin is an antibiotic missile. When it is hurled at other microorganisms, they are shot down by anti-penicillin missiles. What is this anti-penicillin missile?

The Penicillin antibiotic molecule has a beta-lactam ring structure. I do not expect readers to know what a beta-lactam ring is, nor will I delve into its organic chemistry. It suffices to state that a Penicillin antibiotic molecule is torn apart by an enzyme called beta-lactamase (which literally means destroyer of the beta-lactam ring) produced by Penicillin-targeted organisms.

This makes the Penicillin antibiotic lose its potency and allows target organisms to escape the fury of Penicillin.

This is an example of an antibiotic-resistance mechanism. There are many other ways microbes defend against enemy missiles. Another mechanism was already discussed—the strategy of pumping out toxic antibiotics using efflux pumps. I also said the efflux pump principle is a common method wisely used by many lifeforms to get rid of toxic chemicals found in their environment.

Antibiotic molecules are one such toxin that can be dealt with by the pumping action.

Quorum Sensing inhibitors are another class of anti-microbial substances made by plants.

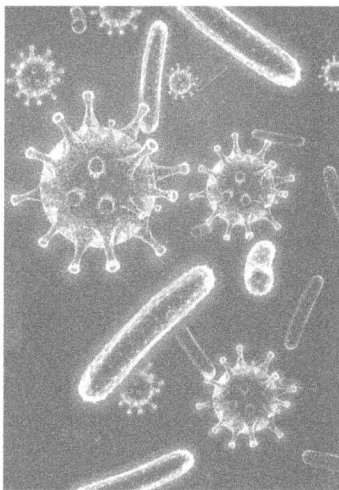

Chapter 9

ANTIBIOTIC RESISTANCE MENACE: MICROBES REVOLT AGAINST ANTIBIOTICS

I AM BASICALLY saying that antibiotics are billions-of-years-old biotechnologies developed by microbes. Anti-antibiotic technology is also billions of years old. We humans learned to use the billions-of-years-old antibiotic technology for our own medical use by targeting these antibiotics at the microbes that infected us.

These microbes are not just in the wild but have entered human territory (i.e., the human body). To fight them, there is no need to re-invent the wheel. Nature did that already. It has ready-made, customized anti-microbial molecules we can use. Billions of years ago, a microbe developed technology for killing bacteria growing in its vicinity and competing for resources.

We use the same antibiotics to kill the same microbes, but call it modern medicine, or pharmacology or whatever. When microbes used these antibiotics for billions of years, it was biological warfare and survival of the fittest. Now, in our eyes, it's modern medicine.

What is happening now? The defense mechanisms evolved by microbes against the antibiotics haunts us in the medical field in the form of the antibiotic resistance phenomenon which the World Health Organization (WHO) described as the biggest challenge faced by modern medicine. Our antibiotics are unable to act as effectively as they should because the target microbes are fighting back with their primal technology.

Now, antibiotic resistance is the biggest threat facing humanity according to WHO. Quickly, our antibiotics are becoming impotent. Bacteria find ways of dealing with antibiotic missiles using all sorts of evasive mechanisms.

I work in a hospital diagnostic laboratory. It is a routine part of our job to test samples collected from infected patients to see what type of microbial organism is growing in their samples—which means identifying the source of their infection. Once the organism is identified, the next step is to check for antibiotic sensitivity.

For this, the organism isolated from the patient is exposed to commonly used antibiotics to see which can kill the bacteria. Based on the lab report, the doctor can choose the right antibiotic for the patient. This practice helps doctors make informed decisions about the antibiotic to be used.

If one were to use any antibiotic they like, chances are the organism might be insensitive to it and while you think you have acted on the microbial source of the patient's infection the microbe inside the patient's body might flourish.

The result will be worsening the disease or even causing death.

Invariably, most of the microbes growing in patients will be insensitive to at least a few of the antibiotics, but we never see microorganisms insensitive to all antibiotics. On the other hand, it is common to see microbes resistant to every antibiotic we tested—we call them Pan Drug-resistant microbes. That is a scary lab report. You are telling the doctor that his or her patient is growing a microbe that will not respond to any antibiotic! Just imagine what would happen if that strain of bacteria started spreading to other patients and to the wider community. That bacteria would be invincible, wouldn't it!

Popular media refers to antibiotic resistant bacteria as Super bugs. They always want catchy titles. What would *you* call a bacterium that defies our medical arsenal?

Antibiotic resistance is a medical term. We specifically refer to medicines used to treat bacterial infections. This term does not apply to viruses because antibiotics do not work against viruses. If you look at nature, all sorts of strategies are used by various lifeforms to fight microbes.

We humans are not the only life systems wanting to ward off hazardous microbes. Most multicellular life forms are susceptible to microbial infections of all sorts. We have the benefit of medical sciences to fight them, but what do the other lifeforms use?

I mentioned Quorum Sensing inhibitors used by plants to kill the microbes infecting them. That is their answer to the problem, but that is not the only answer they have. They make several antimicrobial substances used for their defense against microbes—which we conveniently exploit as well.

I mentioned the medicinal value of turmeric, ginger, neem and so on.

Antibiotic resistance is a capability drawn upon only when needed. Bacteria do not need it all the time. Resistance loses effectiveness if microbes are not exposed to the antibiotics for a long time. It is like our learned skills; if we don't practice a skill, then we become rusty, don't we? We can also totally forget the skill.

Bacteria have just a single cell to operate their life. A lot of life programs are packed in their tiny DNA. It does not have the luxury of multicellular life forms like us where we have a lot of DNA storage space. Even in our digital life, what do we do? Don't we delete files and programs that are not regularly used? We do the same in our cupboards and storage shelves. We throw out things we don't want.

When we isolate a bacterial pathogen from a patient, a

proportion of the bacteria have intact antibiotic resistance skill while others forgot the skill.

So, what happens?

The bacterial population that does not remember how to fight the antibiotics dies. Those that do remember, escape the attack. Sometimes the bacterial population still residing in the patient are predominantly the ones resistant to the antibiotic.

Some bacteria are still left that do not have antibiotic resistance capability. Then, something very interesting happens.

The bacteria possessing antibiotic resistance genes transfer this information to fellow bacteria that do not have them. This is delivered via couriers called Bacteriophages which are viruses that infect bacteria.

When these viruses exit the infected bacteria that happened to have the antibiotic resistance gene, there is a chance those genes are carried along to the next bacteria that they infect.

Antibiotic resistance genes can also be injected into the bacteria during mating between bacteria which is called conjugation. And there is another bizarre way antibiotic resistance genes can transfer between bacteria. When a bacterium dies, its DNA in the form of a strand is liberated outside the cell.

This DNA strand from the dead bacteria is not really dead because its information content is still intact. Amazingly, bacteria can suck free-floating DNA strands from the environment and paste them into their own DNA. The information contained in the sucked-up DNA strand is converted to useable form. If free-floating DNA from the dead bacterium contained antibiotic resistance genes, then the bacteria receiving this lifeless strand of DNA can benefit in a way no different from our software updates.

Can you believe that?

One challenge we face in our modern society is that antibiotics are not only used by us in our hospitals, but they are also widely used in poultry and animal farms.

To prevent infections in chickens and other animals, antibiotics added to their feeds are used in a prophylactic manner.

What is the consequence of this practice?

This means bacteria are often exposed to these antibiotics—which make them acquire antibiotic resistance skills from their fellow bacteria.

If we did not use antibiotics in such farms, the antibiotic resistance phenomenon would be far more manageable.

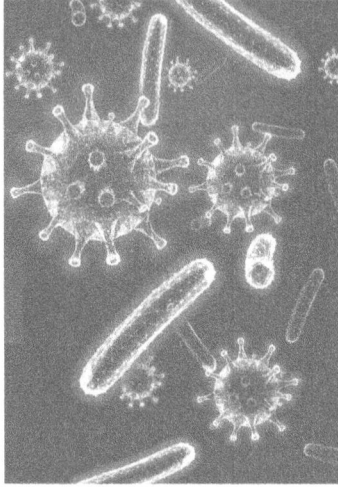

Chapter 10

THE IMMORTALITY OF MICROBIAL INFORMATION

UNICELLULAR LIFE SYSTEMS like bacteria and viruses communicate and exchange information between them and their hosts (or target organisms) using DNA or RNA.

In computer parlance, DNA or RNA are like executable code. We humans never use DNA or RNA in transfer of information except during cell division. Executable codes are not suitable for day-to-day exchange of information in multicellular life forms as they corrupt the genetic code.

This is because different types of cells in multi-cellular life forms use different sets of gene codes in a cell-specific, differential manner (though their full genetic complement is the same in all cells). Use of DNA in cellular information transfers will alter the status of the cells. Viruses damage humans exactly for this reason. Insertion of their DNA or RNA into human cells leads to attachment to human DNA code sequences altering our gene blueprint.

Even viruses that don't attach their codes to human DNA use the host cellular machinery to decipher and execute their executable viral codes. This invariably leads to subversion of the host cells.

Microbe death is very different than complex, multicellular lifeform death. Animals and plants can die of physical trauma, but microbes cannot be beaten or crushed to death.

Microbes are immortal. Left alone, with food and water, microbes can indefinitely divide into daughter cells. They never stop. But our cells do not multiply indefinitely. After about 40-60 cell division cycles, our cells grind to a halt and do not multiply anymore. This is called the Hayflick limit. Our cells are programmed to die. Bacteria and viruses do not have this limit.

Only our germ cells never die. They propagate by meiotic cell divisions. I mean they do not die on their own but can be killed by external forces. The same applies to bacteria and viruses as well.

DNA codes are immortal. Even after millions of years, they can hold information. In the much-acclaimed Steven Spielberg movie *Jurassic Park*, the scientist uses a mosquito trapped in amber for millions of years. That mosquito apparently sucked the blood of the dinosaur that lived 70 million years ago. The scientist extracts the DNA from the dinosaur's blood cells that resided in the mosquito's gut for that long. The idea is that DNA is immortal if it is not physically damaged. This idea is not outlandish.

Some microbes can prolong their life indefinitely. Under harsh environmental conditions, like water and food scarcity, they program their life into a dormant state. Then, the microbe exists in an intermediate state between death and life. It is neither death nor life. It is a state closer to death than to life.

This unusual biological state is called sporulation. Bacterial species like Bacillus and Clostridium, and even some fungal species, can form spores to stay alive indefinitely. In principle, this is like Polar bears going into hibernation during the winter. By hibernating, the polar bear reduces its energy consumption to bare minimum and uses body fat energy for 6 months. Like that, the bacteria and fungi lower their running energy costs to very low levels.

In the year 2000, a team of researchers from West Chester University reported in the journal Nature a startling finding. In a salt pond in the New Mexico region, they identified a bacterial spore dated to be 25 million years old! Once these spores were exposed to water and nutrients they came back to life as if time stood still for them.

25 million years is a long time. Homo sapiens split from the Chimpanzees about 7 million years ago. So, this bacterium lived long before the Homo species originated and long before even Chimpanzees had evolved. For that to happen, the DNA of the bacteria should be intact. This also means the information held by the DNA codes must have been intact too. This is truly amazing. Microbes perfected the technology of preservation of biological matter and biological information to a level we cannot fathom.

Science fiction films talk of space travel by allowing astronauts to hibernate so they will not consume food for long periods. In addition, space travel to faraway stars takes a long time—longer than an astronaut's normal life span. This idea remains fictitious, but microbes achieved this feat.

Scientists analyzing the spores found that the bacteria use a preservative substance called Dipicolinic acid to defy death.

Bacterial spores are a menace to the medical community. They hide in medical instruments and laundry used in the hospitals. If they are not properly destroyed, they can easily spread from patient to patient. To kill the spores, hospitals use sterilization methods that employ temperatures above 120 degrees centigrade for prolonged durations.

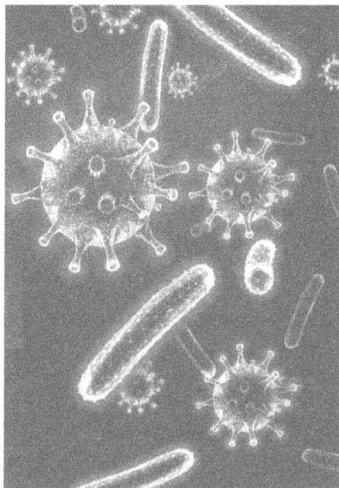

Chapter 11

VIRUSES ARE LIKE BIOLOGICAL TERRORISTS

TERRORISM IS A modern-day phenomenon. In the last few decades, it has grown all over the world. Nations spend a fortune fighting terrorism. They spend a lot of resources on intelligence operations. They track down terrorist movement by maintaining a constant vigil.

I argue that viruses are in every sense of the word like terrorists, so we need to do biological surveillance. We need to track known microbial offenders and try to find ones we do not yet know about. Our nations place a lot of emphasis on counter-intelligence measures against terrorist outfits. They spend a lot of money and resources on it, especially the USA.

Terrorism itself is a new phenomenon in the world. It did not exist in our society as recently as 50 years ago. Whatever the ideology, we geared up to fight these killers all over the world. In my opinion, terrorism is like a pandemic—there are a lot of similarities. Terrorists hit to kill. Viruses and bacteria do the same. The microbes and terrorists do not like to let people live peacefully. Microbial attacks are biological terrorism.

In the same way I say terrorist movements are like social pandemics.

The comparison of viral and bacterial pandemics to terrorist outbreaks is fully justified. Both have the potential to spread quickly. Both can cause devastation when in reality no one gains anything. Will the Corona virus gain something by killing humans en masse? Will it inherit the earth or something? Then why is doing it? The same type of questions can be asked of the terrorists, whatever their ideology and wherever they operate.

Apart from causing fear and panic (which viral pandemics also cause) can terrorist show any real gains? Will putting a few bombs here and there give them anything positive, solve their grievances or promote their ideology?

Another similarity between microbial pandemics and terrorist outbreaks is that they are never permanent. They come and go. They won't bother you all the time, at least not the same microbes and the same terrorist groups. Al Qaida was a social pandemic that hit us in the 1990s. After terrorizing us for over 20 years or so, it finally vanished. It may still operate in some form or other in some countries, but no one talks of them. Then ISIS took over as the next social pandemic causing devastation in the Middle East and other countries too.

United efforts by nations largely incapacitated this terrorist outfit. There have been many other terrorist outbreaks over the years—they come and go. I say the same thing for microbial epidemics. They come and go. We need to accept both as part of our lives. Both will show their ugly faces every now and then.

One more remarkable similarity between social terrorism and biological terrorism is the fact that they can lie low as sleeper cells. These sleeper cells can come alive at unexpected times. There have been viruses and bacteria quietly residing inside human cells for years. The Hepatitis virus (the virus that causes jaundice) can stay alive inside the liver cells for decades. TB bacteria can live inside our lung cells and macrophages for years.

Our experience in fighting terrorism shows that the more the surveillance, the fewer terrorist attacks. There is a clear and positive correlation. Surveillance and counter measures make it much harder for terrorists to carry out attacks. The same principle applies to biological surveillance. If we beef up the search and attack strategy against microbes, you are likely to prevent major disasters like COVID-19.

It is easy to argue against the plan to study and catalog all microbes on the planet on the flimsy ground that many, if not most of them, will never infect humans. Be my guest if you take that position. Also, prepare for global lockdowns and economic turmoil and don't complain. Even COVID-19 virus was supposed to be a zoonotic virus infecting bats and some other animals. Apparently, they made the transition to human hosts due to mutations. It should be possible to identify similar viruses and keep an eye on them or find solutions for fighting them.

I have a question for those who feel it is not cost-effective or practical to study all microbes out there in nature. It could cost a couple of tens of billions of dollars at the most. Pooled money from contributors could be allocated to universities and they will do the rest.

Those who object to this idea should note that all nations put together spent 1,917 billion US dollars in the year 2019 on defense. That is almost 2 trillion dollars in a year. The US alone spent 732 billion dollars, China another 261 billion and India 71 billion. Just three countries amount to a trillion dollars.

What did we use 2 trillion dollars for? We didn't spend this money to alleviate poverty, hunger and disease. We spent this money to fight fellow humans and create destruction. Can you even believe that? It is weird that we are the only life system that spends resources of this magnitude to fight fellow members of the same species.

Most life systems have defense mechanisms of all kinds, requiring a lot of resources, but their efforts are directed against the enemy life forms and not against their own kind. Now we have the audacity to feel bitter about the COVID-19 crisis.

We spent a whopping 70 billion US dollars in 2019 for space exploration. While we were busy exploring and cataloguing stars and black holes millions of light years away, a tiny microbe at our own doorstep wreaked havoc. Did we fail to realize that it is more relevant and important to catalogue microbes in our backyards rather than counting and naming stars and black holes millions of light years away?

With this legacy, my argument for allocating resources to keep an eye on our microbial enemies is difficult to counter. I am pretty sure we could fathom viral mechanisms if only we devoted more resources and attention to it. I cannot believe man will struggle to cope with changing viral mutations and find ways to overcome them. We understand so much about the mechanics of stars and galaxies.

Smart Astrophysicists tell us an asteroid will pass by the earth in 7 million years! They also tell us that 70 million years ago, an asteroid hit our earth leading to the extinction of the dinosaurs! We know much about the parallel universes. The list goes on and on. Sadly, we forgot to look at our own garden. When we were busy looking at the stars, we forgot to study our viral enemies surrounding us.

Lack of surveillance of terrorists costs humanity a lot. In the same way, our inadequate surveillance of microbes costs us even more.

Our internal body is very shrewd. It has an elaborate internal microbial surveillance program constituted by the immune system. What we lack outside our body is compensated by what we are endowed with inside our body. The internal surveillance system is the result of tens of thousands of years of evolution and surely it is bound to be better, smarter and slicker.

I cannot say the same thing about our external world surveillance of microbes. We only know about microbes for the past 200 years or so after we invented the microscope. Even then it takes a lot of time to study each microbe (that we know of).

Scientists study medically important microbes more than others. There is not enough coordination between countries to even think of a global alliance for this purpose. Our internal immune system employs white blood cells as their secret service agents and soldiers: two in one. The ability of our white blood secret service cells in microbial espionage is stupendous. The CIA and FBI pale in comparison to the intelligence operations of white blood cells.

Our body is built like a fort with many levels of checks. Any microbe that wants to enter the human body fort must pass through many layers of biological security checks. Our skin itself is like a wall preventing free entry of external life systems. If it is intact, the skin is an impenetrable wall. If the skin is breached due to an injury, the gap becomes an attractive opportunity for ever present microbes lurking all around.

They try to sneak in. When a wound becomes infected (with microbes), then pus forms around it. The pus is dead white cells who lost their life trying to guard that gaping hole in the skin fortress. In some cases, the microbe may succeed in entering the body and can spread far and wide through the blood stream. A pathogen entering blood can cause serious problems for us. It is called sepsis and is a life-threatening condition.

White blood cells scan for unwanted intruders and do a risk analysis. A dangerous offender with a history of previous intrusions will immediately be known. White blood cells have a microbial crime database they use to check the background of the intruding microbe. A special agent class of white blood cells exists called the Memory cells. These cells have a long memory. Even after decades, they do not forget an offender. They jump into action when they spot a previous offender—even if that microbe offended decades before.

Microbes spot a weakened host easily. If a host is engaged in too many battles, then its army is likely to be depleted. If a person is weak due to poor nutrition, then he or she will not produce ammunition to fight the microbial army.

Frequent or a recent debilitating infection takes a toll on the immune system. In cases like an AIDS infection, the culprit microbe deliberately hits our cellular defenders called CD4 and CD8 cells. This makes it easy for subsequent infecting microbes to enter the body with little resistance. These are called opportunistic infections and that is why AIDS patients frequently get affected by infections.

A war-torn nation is an easy target for external and internal threats. They will easily fall. A country torn apart by internal strife is easy prey for outside enemies. This is like a person with weak immunity who finds it hard to fight microbes like Corona. A person with strong immunity has no problem in beating the microbe.

ISIS was a terrorist pandemic that hit the Middle East, especially around Syria and Iraq, because these nations were debilitated by ongoing, prolonged internal strife that left its army and police very weak and incapable of effective surveillance of dangerous elements.

In the same way, Al Qaida emerged as a pandemic some time ago in Afghanistan because that region was a constant battleground for US and Russian military conflicts.

What caused the world to fall victim to the Corona pandemic? Are we weak as a life system? The problems were related to lack of surveillance. We did not have a robust warning system that would have alerted us earlier. We are weak against viruses. This is due to lack of any effective cure against them.

We also do not know about all the viruses that exist on the planet and naturally have no clue about how to treat them. This is our fault for the reasons I mentioned before. Though we have been hit many times by virus pandemics in the last century, we did not bother to develop anti-viral therapies.

I do not think viruses are cleverer than us. In addition, our societies are concentrated in population—making it easy for microbes to quickly spread far and wide. Maybe viral and bacterial epidemics are natural, self-regulating, cybernetic, feedback mechanisms to curtail a population that grew beyond control.

Microbial epidemics like plague, cholera and influenza occur when living conditions get bad due to overcrowding and a consequent fall in sanitary conditions. It is an alarming idea that microbial infections are in-built, population-control strategies used by Mother Nature.

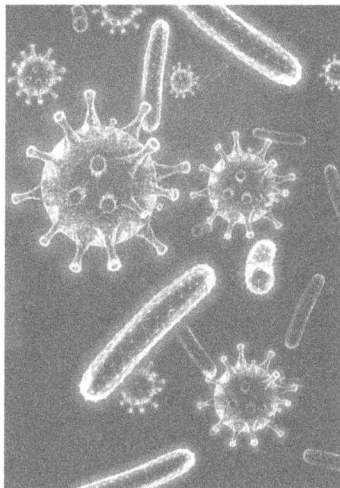

Chapter 12

ARE VACCINES OUR BEST BATTLE STRATEGY AGAINST THE CORONA VIRUS?

AROUND THE WORLD, people eagerly waited for a COVID vaccine to be our ultimate savior. The worldwide public fear led to fast-tracked vaccine efforts around the globe. Weighing the perceived risks against the perceived benefits, governments took extraordinary steps to allow vaccines to be rolled out without the conventional safety studies. Fearing side effects, a significant proportion of the population were reluctant to take these vaccines. Even now, there are many people around the world who are reluctant to take the vaccines.

Pharmaceutical companies and other profit-making organizations reaped financial windfalls from COVID vaccines. Governments were eager to buy them for public health purposes. Countries spent fortunes buying COVID test kits from growing numbers of manufacturers—most situated in China. As I said earlier, private, money-making organizations jumped on the bandwagon. I wish the same zeal and enthusiasm existed earlier for viral surveillance and preparedness.

Countries spent far too much on COVID-related measures using money they did not have. In other words, their debt burden increased—not counting the economic losses due to the lock-down itself. The UK alone is said to have spent about 370 billion pounds as of August 2021 for dealing with COVID and its aftermath. This is just for one viral disease. Just imagine how much could have been gained by the British public if that kind of money was ploughed into NHS to improve collective medical services. What a waste of resources. The same can be said of other nations too.

Little do people know that a vaccine against such respiratory viruses, for example the Flu vaccine, works only in about half of the cases. Only 50-60% of people are truly protected. What is the efficacy rate for COVID vaccines?

Notwithstanding this uncertainty, many organizations rolled out their versions of COVID vaccine. More than 100 such efforts were said to be underway all around the world. It is a good sign, but my question is why didn't we show this urgency in planning before the crisis? What we are doing now is more a desperate attempt to escape from the virus.

One argument against a viral vaccine is the ever-changing structure of the outer wall of the virus. Viruses with low fidelity of replication (accuracy of their copying during replication) end up creating variants soon and often. The COVID virus is said to have undergone at least 200 mutations within the first 6 months of onset. Some of the mutations may have been more detrimental than others. It is also possible in some parts of the world that the types of mutations that happened in their viral strains made them less deadly and that is why they were not so much affected in terms of death rates.

Every now and then a news item appears in the media that new strain has been identified in some country and suddenly there is renewed anxiety in the minds of millions of the public. The public health agencies initiate further efforts to deal with the new strain. Just when national lockdowns were being removed all over the world, the new strain called Omicron appeared in South Africa. Despite lack of evidence that it was deadly, the media did their round of publicity and there is again talk of restricted air travel and lockdowns.

Unexpectedly, protests happen in some parts of the world against renewed and continued governmental efforts to restrict public—citing COVID risks—which tells us we might have overreacted to the COVID crisis like our immune system sometimes does, resulting in a defensive protection with pitiably small gain compared to the unwanted damages.

I refer particularly to the Cytokine storm that kills the COVID patients. Lockdowns and other global efforts may have been as damaging—or more damaging—as the virus itself.

One school of thought that existed from the beginning of the pandemic is that lockdowns were unnecessary. There were scientists who felt that COVID infections should have been dealt with as another viral epidemic and to let the herd immunity deal with it. I am sure there are many policymakers and scientists all over the world who silently shared the same idea but got buried by the massive hype built around the problem.

No one can argue against the fact that natural infections stimulate immune defense against multiple antigens on the surface of the COVID virus compared to the vaccine. Vaccines are typically prepared using a single antigen as the stimulus and therefore runs the risk of impotence if that antigen mutates (which is bound to happen).

Every time a new variant of the COVID virus was discovered, the question was asked: will our vaccines still be effective? Scientists repeatedly showed that the build-up of viral antibodies in our system is far more varied and in higher quantities in naturally infected people than in vaccinated people.

The other point to be noted is that there is much talk about the transmissible rate of a Corona virus strain. If it is highly transmissible, then we go through another bout of anxiety and stress thanks to the media. Little do we realize that the faster rate of transmission means that nature is vaccinating large numbers of the public free of cost. This should mean that there will be benefits of herd immunity protecting the population.

Considering the low mortality rate of Corona virus infection—counting on herd immunity is not a bad approach to take. In heavily populated countries with little resources for vaccination or testing, this helped to keep the pandemic under control. If we analyzed infection rates and mortality compared with public spending across all nations, chances are we would be disappointed by the effectiveness of government spending. But, due to morality and ethical issues, there would be a lot of hue and cry if we approached the problem from this angle. However, the common man affected by the economic tsunami will have a different opinion.

My question is: why do vaccine researchers always target the outer coat of the virus? Why doesn't anyone look at aiming at the interior of the virus? The interior of the virus is conserved and not much changes there. Mutations do not affect the interior structure or process of the virus. I read a news item recently about a research group looking at hitting the inside of the virus—not the outside—and they were very excited about it.

Why didn't the scientific community think of this a long time ago for other viruses? Are we paying the price for our negligence? The price is surely high.

Spanish Flu hit us early in the 20th century and killed 50-70 million people. In just 6 months, 25 million people were dead. One might say we are not as advanced scientifically and medically. Moreover, we were too preoccupied with our pastime, i.e., war. Hardly anything was done against the Spanish Flu from a scientific point of view.

Recently, there were many pictures circulating in social media showing people living during that time wearing masks just like us. Apparently, there were lockdowns of schools and theaters even those days. What surprises me is that when COVID-19 virus hit us there was conflicting advice regarding the use of masks in prevention. Even WHO stated that the masks helped only symptomatic people from contaminating others.

Masks were also advised only for healthcare personnel who were in contact with suspected or infected patients. There was no advice at that time favoring the use of masks by the general public. Isn't it common sense that masks will likely halt the virus from spreading to others? Didn't we do that during the Spanish Flu? Then why wasn't the mask made compulsory right from the beginning? I feel it could have helped in a big way.

One curious consequence of people wearing masks, adopting social distancing and closing of schools, etc. is that other common respiratory infections largely subsided! We notice this in hospitals. We do not see those patients anymore. It is a definite trend. There is a drastic reduction in other respiratory infections thanks to the safety measures we took for COVID.

That benefit comes from an unexpected quarter. Not all microbes, known or unknown, are killers. There are grades of severity in the ways they interact with us. First, not all microbes can infect humans. When it comes to infections, there is species-specific affinity for certain life systems. A microbe that infects a bird may not have the know-how to infect humans. A microbe infecting a plant might be harmless towards a human. The viruses that hit other animals (other than man) are known as Zoonotic viruses. Every form of animal life system will have its own share of these troublemakers.

Where we are susceptible to a microbe, generally the consequences of an infection can be harmless or even beneficial. The next level of effect could be a mild infection like a common cold. Some microbes have more impact and can cause troubling and long-lasting infections. It could be pneumonia, brain fever (encephalitis), or infections of organs like kidney, liver, bone etc.

These will often require a hospital admission. An extreme form of an infection could cause death. I suppose one could liken the grades of severity of microbial infections to the range of social outcasts. You could see a harmless beggar on the street. There could be unruly kids on the streets causing minor damage to property or people. Then there are gangs known to be low lives. Their job is to terrorize the neighborhood and indulge in drugs, burglary and gang wars. Above this will be criminals who live a life of thievery and crime—they are the ones who get the attention of the police force, and all sorts of measures are taken to curb them. Above these local criminals, we have the mafia that operates on a widescale—they are feared more than local criminals because of their ruthlessness. The extreme end of the spectrum are the terrorist outfits whose sole mission is to create death and destruction. They can cause social pandemics. They are like microbial pandemics requiring global action. That is what happened with COVID 19.

It is obvious the retaliation to a microbial attack will depend on its nature and consequence. Out of the 6,500 viruses known to man now (including the 6,300 that do not infect man) there are common properties between them. This helped us classify them into 25 families. Viruses grouped into families behave similarly—they have common characteristics.

It's like classifying humans according to religion, nationality, caste, creed and so on. Even terrorist outfits can be categorized into distinct types based on their ideology. Microbial classes, not only the viruses but including bacteria, are countered by measures unique to their type and infectious characteristics. Surveillance goes a long way in ascertaining the nature of an offending microbe.

Often, moderately dangerous microbes continuously challenge mankind and possibly other life systems. They don't hit in pulses. They are there all the time. Some microbes hit in a big way every now and then. They cause outbreaks and epidemics. When they reach a global scale, we call them Pandemics.

Bacteria like Vibrio Cholera (the bacteria that causes Cholera pandemic), Salmonella (the bacteria that causes Typhoid), and Yersinia pestis (the bacteria that causes the dreaded bubonic plague) cause big outbreaks in a periodic manner.

Viruses like the Flu virus, SARS, MERS, COVID-19, Hantan, Ebola, Nipah and Zika viruses appear suddenly and hit us badly. COVID-19 was bad not least due to its virulence but due to panic manufactured by the media.

We need global cooperation to form an alliance tasked with microbial surveillance. This should have been our strategy from the beginning. This should be a collective effort by all humanity and should be supported by national governments and rich multinational corporations. One could even make it mandatory for such rich companies to make annual contributions for the Global Alliance on Microbial Surveillance.

When COVID-19 hit our global economy, many businesses and industries were deeply affected. Now they want the government to bail them out. If we had the vision to think of a collective effort to watch for hazardous microbes, then we would not be suffering now. We should study and build a database of all microbes—irrespective of whether they attack humans or not.

Microbes can frequently jump species barriers ever and a typical Zoonotic virus can become capable of infecting man too. This new ability is gained by the virus or bacteria because of random mutation or when they gain access to man in the form of food. Chinese have the habit if eating many creatures including snakes, bats, monkeys etc. This enables microbes infecting such animals to find their way into humans. Once in, perhaps they then figure out a way to colonize mankind.

Global cooperation toward health improvement is the remit of the World Health Organization. This non-profit body has the laudable goal of improving the health and well-being of people living on the planet. They need financial contributions from member countries to make this happen.

At a time of greatest need, the US government withdrew support to WHO—which might be counter-productive. Nations should be more visionary than that. We should move away from such disruptive strategies and build more powerful alliances supported by public and private enterprises. This should not only be just the domain of government.

Most countries operate on deficit budgets. One should not be optimistic that national leaders will have the care and understanding to contribute monetary support for microbial surveillance. That is why I think a joint enterprise is necessary— with private corporations who are eager to pounce on profit-yielding ventures, but shy away from social responsibilities. They are more interested in measuring revenue. Apple became the first two-trillion-dollar company in the world. To date, Amazon is slightly short of a two-trillion valuation.

We count the world's rich where the top 100 people have at least a few billion each. A social responsibility tax should be levied on rich individuals and companies to help fund initiatives such as global microbial surveillance.

This effort should catalog all forms of bacteria and viruses and conduct a search for combat measures appropriate for each of the dangerous ones.

If we remain complacent, like we have always been, be my guest. Expect to be hit hard every so often. Growing populations, increasing population density and the ease of air travel will make infectious outbreaks happen more frequently.

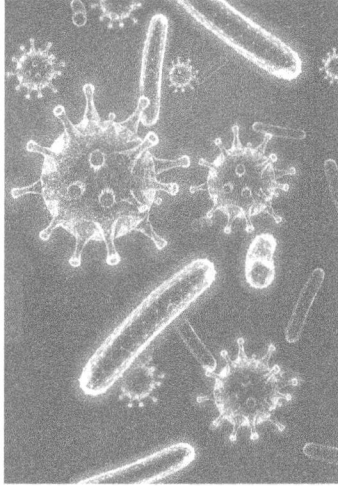

Chapter 13

VIRAL INFECTIONS ARE LIKE CYBERCRIMES

THE CORONA VIRUS, like other viral enemies, adopts a battle strategy aimed at exhausting us rather than fighting head-on. Viruses cannot win a battle played by textbook rules. Slyness is required to win against a massive enemy like us. That is why they hit our lungs and make us incapable of fighting back. Why do our body defense soldiers (white blood cells) fail to identify and destroy these culprits? I ask the same question about all types of microbes that manage to give the slip to our body's internal surveillance mechanisms. The reason is: these microbes hack our body like cybercriminals!

Can you believe that?

I argue that real viruses are like computer viruses to the letter. This is the first time anyone compared a real virus to a computer virus—instead of vice versa.

Real viruses are executable codes injected into our cells to carry out functions against the wish of the host cells. They are forced instructions to do things that benefit the virus and can be harmful to the host. Operating systems of living systems are based on either DNA or RNA. Life systems use A (Adenine), T (Thymine), G (Guanine) and C (Cytosine) as the quaternary digits no different from what the binary digits (0 and 1) used in our computers and other digital devices.

Our operating system runs many cellular applications like computer Apps. These days, there are millions of different computer Apps (Applications) running a variety of functions. The word App is now an integral part of our social lives. Little do we realize that our own body has Apps too.

We have an App for digestion, an App for breathing, an App for excretion, an App for thinking, an App for movement, an App for vision, an App for hearing, an App for reproduction and so on. They are all controlled by our DNA operating system like the computer operating system running our computer applications.

These cellular Apps are executed by codes written in DNA language using the ATGC digits. God wrote these body programs like IT professionals write the computer programs.

Viruses, including Corona, have executable code that helps them hack into one of our cellular applications. To do that, their executable codes can subvert the host's defense. A usual ploy of a virus is to mimic a host molecule to gain unauthorized entry. All sorts of viruses and bacteria evolved strategies to enter the host by camouflage. Computer viruses and worms do the same. They come into our phones or computers via an innocuous message or email and anyone who clicks and opens them thinking they are genuine messages or emails execute the codes concealed in that message which unleash a variety of harmful outcomes.

Most often, computer hackers want to access your personal details and bank account passwords, etc. If a hacker aims at an organization, he will look toward entering their control sites to cause chaos. In 2004, the My Doom computer virus infected 250,000 computers in one day (the same rate of COVID-19 virus infection rate on a global scale). In 2007, the I Love You computer virus infected over 50 million computers in a span of about 8 months from January to October. Way back in 1999, the

Melissa computer virus accessed our computers in the disguise of an email. Major corporations—including Microsoft—had to lockdown their email servers like COVID-19 virus accessed our Breathing App and led to the lockdown of the entire planet!

Corona's master plan is like that of a James Bond film Villain. Like real life terrorist attacks or in movies, the villain attacks where it hurts. They never choose a small-time target simply because the impact will not be there. Viruses like Corona do indeed have a mega-budget plan.

The Corona virus conducted a cybercrime attack on humanity. It is not unique in that respect as all viruses are information hackers. The Corona virus hacked into our breathing App by gaining unlawful entry mimicking the human ACE2 protein. The ACE2 receptor on lung cells in our body unwittingly opens their gates when the Corona virus comes near them—thinking it is an ACE2 molecule.

This is called natural mimicry, an evolutionary ploy many life systems adopt. This is like stealing someone's password, PIN number or passport to gain unlawful access. That is what hackers and criminals do.

What is the Corona virus trying to achieve by doing this? One can understand a terrorist or a thief trying this kind of unlawful, disguised entry as they stand to achieve monetary or ideological benefit. But what does this tiny Corona virus gain by doing this and ultimately killing us?

Nowadays cybercrimes are not only the territory of criminals. Some nations chose this as a war strategy. Nations deliberately plan digital attacks on enemy nations and create havoc. This is a cheap and effective method of hurting your enemy. It is a low-cost weapon.

For tiny life systems which do not have a massive biological infrastructure, this kind of attack on enemy operating systems (or cellular applications) is cost-effective and practical. Largely, tiny life systems like microbes adopt this method as a means of attacking their multicellular hosts. They are never equals but can wreak havoc like the Corona virus did. Microbes conduct biological warfare using cyber tactics.

I accuse microbes of being cybercriminals. Have I justified my claim?

Let's look at some other viruses.

The Polio virus hits us at our communication towers to interfere with transmission of biological information across nerve cables. Ganglions are nerve communication interchanges situated all along the spinal cord which is the information highway of our body. All sorts of commands are sent by the brain to different body parts down this spinal cord information highway.

What do these Polio viruses do? They attack the ganglion cells in the spinal cord and interfere with the transmission of information from the brain to the muscles. The brain loses its ability to command the muscle cells to initiate or terminate movement. That is why the Polio victims are paralyzed or have severe weakness of limbs.

Messages coming from the brain are intercepted by the polio viruses just like criminals destroy the communication towers or the telecommunication cables. The Polio virus, in short, hacks into our command center and the information exchange points. Where did the Polio virus study Electronics and Communications engineering? I don't understand why the Polio virus wants to hack into our spinal cord App and cut-off the communication channels from the brain to the lower part of the body. Here, I see only pointless, evil desire. The Polio virus has largely been eradicated from our planet thanks to a vaccine. Very few sporadic cases are seen nowadays. It is no longer a threat to us.

The virus that causes brain fever (Encephalitis) is another deadly cybercriminal. It infects brain neurons and causes inflammation. Nerve connections between nerve cells are damaged. Nerve cells in the brain are the equivalent of a single computer. There are billions of nerve cells in the brain making it the largest Internet in the Universe. There is a lot of information flowing to and fro in these brain cell connections forming the basis of our body functions like thinking, talking, hearing, and a whole lot of other higher functions. If these brain internet connections are disrupted, brain activity descends into chaos. The encephalitis virus does damage like cybercriminals who hack the Internet.

Jaundice is a layman's term denoting damage caused by a virus inflaming the liver. It is medically called Hepatitis. There are many types of Hepatitis viruses, but the types B and C are the more damaging. There is no effective cure for the Hepatitis viruses in Allopathic medicine. This does not mean we have cures for other viruses, but for Hepatitis virus—we have nothing. We do not have effectives cure for any type of virus—including the common cold virus. There is no doubt about it; we are very weak against our viral enemies. That is why we were hit so hard by the Corona virus.

Viruses generally target a single organ. They are incapable of infecting all the organs in the body. This is because their know-how of hacking into a host animal is limited to one organ system. Hepatitis viruses can only infect the liver cells and no other types of cells. These viruses have gene programming to hack and inactivate the Liver App of our body. Our bodies' Liver App is an important one. Like the Corona virus targeting our breathing App, the hepatitis virus targets our Liver App.

The liver is like the industrial organ of the body. There are many essential molecules manufactured in the liver and if the liver is damaged, then the body suffers due to the absence of a number of these molecular products. This includes plasma proteins and clotting factors for example.

Apart from the manufacturing job, the liver is central to protein metabolism. The waste product of the protein metabolism, ammonia, is toxic to the brain. If left unchecked, ammonia can cause coma. This is called a hepatic coma—a serious medical condition. The liver helps us avoid this in our daily lives by converting the toxic ammonia into harmless urea which is then excreted in the urine.

This vital function is affected if the hepatitis virus attacks the liver. Due to this, patients are unable to handle simple dietary proteins. That is why patients with jaundice are forbidden from consuming proteins in their diet.

The Liver App also has a detoxification function. Daily, we are all exposed to all sorts of environmental pollutants, including from food additives, coloring agents and/or the medicines we take. We are exposed to industrial pollutants. These foreign molecules are detoxified by the Liver App by means of an extensive system of enzymes. If we lose this capacity like a jaundice patient, toxic chemicals can cause unchecked damage.

The liver also is important for packaging our dietary fat in the form of lipoproteins absorbed from the gut. A jaundiced patient cannot do this and therefore is unable to handle dietary fat. This is why jaundiced patients are not allowed to eat fatty foods.

The liver is also the site where blood clotting factors are made. These clotting factors are protein molecules and there are many types of them. They are functionally arranged in the form of a cascade. For blood to clot (like in a bleeding scenario) the topmost clotting factor must first be activated which then activates the next clotting factor and so on. This activation is sequentially passed down the cascade until the last member of the clotting factor is activated which then leads to a clot that will plug the leaking blood vessel.

If this clotting cascade is unnecessarily activated. then the blood will clot for no reason. This can cause a blood flow blockage. If that blockage happens in the heart, then it can cause a heart attack. If the blockage happens in the brain, then it can cause a stroke.

So, the clotting function should be tightly controlled. This is the function of the Liver App.

Why do I elaborate so much about the liver function? How is it relevant here? The reason why I described liver function in detail is to show that we are going to be hard-hit if a virus like the hepatitis virus hacks into the Liver App. It is amazing to think that the hepatitis virus knows what a strategic target the liver is.

How does Cholera cause such swift death? Why is it so dangerous? Cholera bacteria produces a chemical toxin that attacks the human intestine. Normally, we would describe this as chemical warfare and UN would come running to protest that this is not a just method of warfare. In our society, we decided that chemical warfare is abhorrent. This is strange because we use deadly incendiary arms in war, but somehow chemical warfare is an inhuman method. Anyway, that is beside the point to be discussed here.

Cholera toxin causes water scarcity in our body. We can say it causes drought. Cells dry out. In medical terms, we call this dehydration. Our body has about 40-50 liters of water—water constitutes almost 60% of our body weight. Water is fundamentally important for body metabolism and biochemical reactions come to a halt if we do not have enough water.

Our body conserves water wherever possible. A considerable amount of water purified by the kidney is reabsorbed in kidney tubules. About 1 liter of blood filters through the kidneys each minute. Water being a major constituent of blood, that means, unless the kidney reabsorbs this water, many liters of water could be wasted as urine. But, on average we only excrete about 1-2 liters of water every day as urine. This illustrates the efficiency of water conservation in the body. In the same way, our intestines also have water reabsorption mechanisms in the lower intestine allowing it to conserve water. Just like we save rainwater, our body also saves it.

Thirst sensation is controlled by a sensor at the base of the brain. This sensor detects the water level in the body like we measure water levels in a dam. In our bodies, we need enough water, but not too much of it. Too much is like a harmful flood.

The water balance in our body is run like a computer App or cybernetic system. The cholera toxin hacks the water balance App of our body. How does it do this?

Our lower intestinal water reabsorption system is based on a molecular suction apparatus capable of Open and Shut settings. When needed, this tap can be opened or closed. This molecular suction apparatus is controlled by a particular protein called G Protein. G proteins are versatile molecules playing key roles in surface communication and control on top of each cell. They are stationed on the cell tops—including the intestinal wall cells.

There are so many types of G proteins, and each has a different role to play. One such function of a G protein is to monitor the water tap in the intestine. The Cholera toxin binds the G protein and arm-twists it into the open position. The water in the intestinal cavity leaks through open water channels and exits the body as explosive, watery diarrhea.

Many liters of water can be lost in a short time—enough to create a severe drought in the body. It is like someone bombed your dams to allow saved rainwater to drain away. Cholera toxin is a water dam buster. This deadly microbe came back time and again killing millions of people. I don't understand the motive of this this tiny microbe that has such a grudge against us that it wants us to die of water scarcity.

What a cruel microbe this is.

Life systems evolved survival skills aimed at water conservation. This is even more important in desert regions. To use tactics interfering with water conservation as a method of killing is pretty high-tech. The Cholera microbe uses a high-tech, molecular tool acting like a precision-guided missile that hits our water storage sites. If we were tasked with developing nanotechnology that precisely alters molecular water channels, we would require scientists from top class universities and spend millions of dollars in a big lab. It is mind-boggling to think that the tiny, one-celled cholera bacteria can achieve this with no need for science, big funding or a big lab.

Before I move on, I want to mention a few herbal plants that seem effective against the jaundice virus. These are widely used in India and many other countries. These herbal plants are the anti-virus software for Hepatitis.

Viruses conduct their attacks by targeting host communications and applications such that one or more critically important applications or a command center will be made non-functional. It beats me why they would want to do this. It is unclear what their incentive is. The same strategy is used against all susceptible organisms. They are cyber specialists par excellence.

An amazing thing about viruses is they are not self-sufficient programs. Their executable codes are inadequate for independent living. Their simple DNA or RNA codes are capable of only a few tasks. Invariably, one of these tasks will be an information-based attack on the host using a disguised entry. The viruses can only survive for 2-3 days if they fail to hatch onto a host cell. They need to hitchhike a ride by tagging onto a host operating system. Their own operating system is based on a few code snippets and is inadequate for creating a full-fledged life.

Some viruses—like the HIV virus—enter the host cell and their RNA information codes are converted to DNA codes which are then integrated into the DNA operating system of the human host cell. From then on, the HIV virus programs are run using the human host-cell deciphering tools. Because the viral codes are safely integrated with the host-cell operating system, no retaliation from the host happens.

None of the immune system warriors can even think of attacking the HIV virus because it merged with the host life codes. Incredibly enough, the HIV virus also inactivates the host fighter lymphocytes, and the patient loses the ability to fight the HIV virus.

The inability of fighting microbes does not stop with the HIV virus. Other microbes can infect these patients with ease. A weakened immune system is like a nation weakened due to economic problems, frequent wars and internal strife draining their time and resources. Opportunistic infections become the order of the day. In a country depleted of its resources, invariably, internal factions start rioting and looting which is very similar to the way innocuous microbes gain the upper hand in a weak host and cause major infections.

Viruses are unable to reproduce on their own. For that reason, one can ask whether the viruses are living beings or not? Are they inanimate? Looking at the way they execute cybercrimes by entering the host body like a computer virus or worm, one won't be criticized for suggesting these viruses are inanimate—as inanimate as the real computer viruses. They are just nucleic acid codes written in the quaternary genetic language.

Viruses literally inject their nucleic acid codes into the host cells. Also, bacteria are known to inject raw genetic codes into fellow bacterial cells. This process of transferring nucleic acid codes is called Conjugation when it happens between two bacterial cells. Sometimes, free-floating genetic code strings can be taken up by bacteria, which is called Transformation. This is like computer program code entering by injection!

We, multicellular life forms, rely on various methods for intercellular communication—via hormones, growth factor, neurotransmitter, or cytokine (agents released during infections and inflammations by immune cells). They are mostly proteins in nature.

They could also be even simpler, such as a modified amino acid. An example is Gamma Amino butyric Acid (GABA) which is a widely prevalent neurotransmitter in the nervous system mediating inter-neuronal communications. Sometimes even a simple, unmodified, amino acid can be an informational molecule. A typical example is Glycine.

Multicellular life forms never use their genetic codes directly for intercellular communication. Rather, they use the products of the genetic code. The advantage is that these derived products (derived from the information contained in the genetic code) do not mess with the operating system of the recipient cells. If we used the DNA codes as messages, then the DNA code must first be integrated to the recipient cell operating system which is also DNA. This will tamper with the recipient cell's operating system. Use of executable codes for information transfer between cells is taboo in multicellular life.

Unicellular life forms like microbes use executable, genetic codes only for communication purposes. They use similar executable genetic codes when they infect a host. They deliver an executable code that will be executed by the host-cell machinery. On that basis they are no different from computer viruses and worms that hackers use.

Viruses and bacteria typically have a narrow host spectrum. They cannot infect all types of life systems. This is because their infection strategy will be based on using a particular type of executable code compatible with a particular type of operating system only. For the same reason, no computer virus exists that can infect any operating system. Computer viruses spread easily from one computer to another because most computers use Windows operating system. This creates a monoculture of computers.

In other words, many computers are identical and therefore uniformly susceptible to computer viruses using executable codes compatible with Microsoft Windows. God prevented simultaneous destruction of all life forms by designing unique operating systems in various animals, insects, birds and plants. Otherwise, one virus could hit and destroy all known life forms. God created inbuilt anti-virus protection and he was one hell of a Cyber security expert.

Our current generation of computers uses Windows, Linux and Apple Mac operating systems. A computer virus that hacks one type of operating system cannot infect the other two types. That saves us from being affected en masse. Our phones, which are powerful computers, use Android, IOS (the iPhone operating system), and a host of other minor types of operating systems. They are less prominent species.

When personal computers came about 50-70 years ago, no one knew what a Cybercrime was. As a result, no one knew what Cyber security was. It was not even thought there would be a need to protect digital information. Nobody thought of it.

When financial institutions started using computers, it became apparent that unwanted elements could access your financial data. Customers noticed their data (money) was not safe. They complained to their financial institutions about the lack of security for their money and data.

Financial institutions were themselves customers to the IT companies that made the computers and software. They were not the original designers of online finance. Even IT companies like Microsoft, Apple, and IBM were not prepared for this. They did not anticipate the need for digital protection. Computers after all started as faster calculators. Nobody foresaw that one day they would be used for online banking and other financial transactions.

If we were only using computers for calculations and typing, the hackers would have little interest. But, when computers became widespread and people used them for everything, the hackers saw opportunities. Even apart from financial data, theft hackers stole vital company secrets and other confidential information from important companies and even from government departments.

Defense departments of nations became targets for such malicious attacks. Back in the 1960s and 1970s—and even the 1980s, IT companies were unaware of the need to make computers safe. For them, the money was already made by selling the computers and software and it was of no concern to them that the customers were unsafe.

There was really a period of resistance and lack of interest from computer companies in spending money on computer security. But constant pressure from financial companies made them budge and then many cyber security measures came about.

The anti-virus software that all of us use in our computers is one such cyber security tool.

I suppose our society is new to terrorism too. I do not think terrorist groups existed before about 100 years ago. Our human society is only about 4,000-5,000 years old. Only then did political establishments begin forming. Until then man lived in small tribes. The population of such tribal groups was a few hundred to a few thousand until cities and states started forming 4,000-5,000 years ago.

Slowly, the population of human groups started expanding. That made it necessary for the kings to monitor the subjects by some sort of surveillance mechanism—through spies or other means. This was necessary to thwart thieves and even dissident groups who were unhappy with the king. A tool used to monitor people was creating the fear of God—a low-cost method of making people behave.

Over time, our social surveillance methods became more and more complex. We not only monitor criminal elements, but also enemy nations. Funded by nations, elaborate networks of secret service agencies now operate worldwide. Before 5,000 years ago I do not think our societies needed any form of surveillance. But, over time we have come to need these costly measures to keep our society safe. This is no different from the way IT companies were indifferent in the beginning, but later progressed with anti-virus software, Firewalls and what not.

Life systems face the same need to keep their genetic information safe. Competition from other life forms threatens the continued existence of their genetic information. When a species becomes extinct, their genetic information is lost. But these are rare events.

More common threats come from prey-predator relationships between lifeforms. Intriguing are the relationships of man and other lifeforms with tiny creatures called Microbes. I am unsure about the biological benefit microbes gain by attacking our genetic information. Surely, life systems—including us—evolved a variety of anti-virus strategies and anti-bacterial strategies. Viruses and bacteria seem smart too. They come up with evasive strategies to help them beat our plans.

The immune evasion tactics of microbes are as unbelievable as science fiction.

Some life forms closely related in evolutionary lineage are similar in their operating systems. So, they may be promiscuous and might fall for the attack of the same virus. Children often resemble someone else in the family and even if you do not know them in person, just by observing, you can identify them as a brother, son or father of someone you know. This similarity is due to common DNA codes between them because they are related. Microbes also use DNA similarity to hit related species.

Life systems perhaps are naturally protected by this operating system dependency of viruses and bacteria. That is why the same microbe cannot infect more than a few types of living systems. A virus that hits a plant cannot infect a human because both hosts use different operating systems, and the virus cannot tamper with both. In the same way, a virus that normally infects a chicken or a lion often cannot infect humans.

Viruses that infect animals are called Zoonotic viruses. For some reason, a virus that infects an animal can acquire the ability to infect humans too. This is said to happen by closer interaction of the susceptible animal with man. In China people eat all sorts of animals including bats, insects, snakes and so on. It is possible that a virus infecting these animals can adapt to humans once ingested.

This may not happen quickly.

It may take some time for the virus to hack into humans. For that, they need to steal the password that opens the human body. This password is like a fake passport. Usually, what happens is that the virus integrates itself with human DNA at some point by some means. Then after some time they get detached and separate out again.

When this happens, it is possible that some extra bit of human DNA comes along in the viral nucleic acid. It is like stealing our gene codes. This extra bit of human DNA may remain in the viral operating system and whenever these human codes are deciphered while the viral operating system is running, the product of that bit of human DNA code may be made.

Obviously, because the code came from man, the product looks same as a human molecule in part or full. This similarity is the key to human entry—it allows the virus to steal an entry because our human cellular mechanisms cannot distinguish between the virally made, humanoid molecule (human-like) and the real human molecule. Thus, the viral infiltrator enters the human fortress.

In fact, one of the theories about the origin of viruses postulates that viruses are spilt-over breadcrumbs of human DNA. When you eat a biscuit or a croissant, you spill some crumbs. It is annoying and messy. Theorists put forward the exotic idea that such crumbs falling off your DNA codes during cell divisions or other cell processes had life potential in them because after all they broke off from a life system's operating system.

That life potential bloomed when those crumbs were read by a system. Possible annealing (joining) of such bits of spilt-over gene codes could have led to a meshwork of life codes that formed a prototype virus. That prototype virus (or viruses) may have evolved further by possible code exchanges between them.

The affinity of two strands of gene codes to seek out each other is driven by the chemical structure of gene codes. Adenine (A) will pair with Thymine (T) and Guanine (G) will pair with Cytosine (C). So, the free-floating nucleic acid gene codes may have tried to re-trace their way back to the DNA-holding nucleus of the human cell. I keep referring to this DNA held in the nucleus as the operating system of the cell (or species). That re-tracing step transformed to the phenomenon of infection.

Though the theory described above sounds very exotic it is a legitimate explanation offered for the origin of the viruses in standard textbooks. So, readers should not conclude that I am talking gibberish.

Bacteria can absorb free-floating DNA from dead bacteria and assimilate the information held in it. This is unbelievable. I heard of an African tribe with the custom of eating the brain of the deceased elderly. The reason for this age-old custom was their belief that they would acquire the wisdom of that dead individual. The bacteria seem to think like this tribe.

Bacteria can exchange vital information by the exchange of gene code patches—no different from the way we use software patches. Antibiotic resistance capability is held by some genes in some bacteria. These resistance genes confer the ability to fight the antibiotic and escape their fury. The bacteria give these genes the ability to send copies of these genes to neighbor bacteria that do not have it.

A population of bacteria infecting a human host may contain a mix of species of bacteria that have the antibiotic resistance genes and those that don't. Those that have these genes can offer these gene codes as free-gene code injections or exchange between two conjugating bacteria during the cell division.

The point I emphasize is that viruses can acquire gene codes from a source and use them. Similar to needing computer hardware to run our software, viruses need support machinery to run their gene programs. The Corona virus software is programmed to hack the human breathing App. It is ironic that this software is run by our own cellular hardware. This is where the malevolent intention of the virus comes into focus. It concocted an evil plan and successfully subverted our cellular computers to do what it wants. That is why I liken microbial viruses to computer viruses created by hackers with the sole idea of harm.

I don't understand what the viruses gain by doing this. Hackers might demand ransoms and expect to be paid in Bitcoins. What the virus gains, I do not know. Intriguingly, after the host dies, doesn't the virus end up in the cold again? Isn't it beneficial not to kill the host? Then why kill?

At this juncture I would like to draw attention to the similarities between a terrorist group and the viruses (both biological and computer viruses). I earlier said terrorist outbreaks are like viral pandemics and that for tackling both, a lot of surveillance is required. In both cases, we face a big penalty if there is not enough surveillance and countermeasures.

Some may not agree with this comparison, but that's their opinion. To me, the ideology of a terror group is an executable moral code deliberately fed into people's minds. Once fed, this executable moral code spreads to others too. People subscribing to this terror group will go to some extent to cause havoc.

Moral ideology works exactly like computers and biological viruses—taking over the minds of a large section of our society. At one point, even those who do not subscribe to this ideology get affected and start suffering the consequences. The role of terrorist group leaders is to inject such thoughts into people's minds like computer hackers do.

Bacteria are hackers too. Even fungi are information hackers. They both use information hacking as a means of fighting their competitors. I talk about fellow bacteria that compete for nutrients and resources. Here, I am not referring to infections of animals or humans. I said a while ago that antibiotics are molecules found in nature produced by fungi and some bacteria. They are the battle weapons used to kill enemy microbes. How do these antibiotics kill? Would it surprise you if

I told you that antibiotics are information-targeting hacking tools.

Some antibiotics like Ciprofloxacin belong to the antibiotic class Quinolones and hit the operating system of the microbe i.e., DNA. For the DNA codes to be read and deciphered (something that must happen when the organism performs a life task) the DNA strands must be uncoiled and straightened.

DNA is kept in a highly coiled form twisted around a protein core like the thread is wound around a tailor's spindle. For DNA to be read they must be unwoven in select parts so that the deciphering molecules can act on them. One such unwinding tool is an enzyme called DNA gyrase. This enzyme helps to unwind the DNA. Ciprofloxacin and related antibiotics prevent this DNA from unwinding and blocks the DNA information decoding. The targeted microbes literally die from information starvation. In simple terms, antibiotics kill by preventing enemy microbes from using their own information.

In other words, the makers of these antibiotics (bacteria and fungi) are cybercriminals too.

Antibiotics like Tetracycline are made by the Streptomyces species of Actinobacteria. They attack their enemy bacteria by hitting the DNA translation step. The normal process of decoding DNA information for execution of life tasks requires the information held in the DNA to be translated to a protein form.

First the DNA information is converted to the form of messenger RNA which is basically a string of nucleotide letters like we write computer programs using 0 and 1 binary digits. The only difference is the messenger RNA uses A, T, G and C letters. Moreover, they are read by the cellular apparatus called the ribosomes three letters at a time. Each of these three letters code for insertion of a specific amino acid in the synthesis of proteins which are basically amino acids arranged like letters in a sentence. So, all the 20 amino acids available in nature have a pre-fixed three letter code called the codons. The ribosomes assemble amino acids per the code instruction in messenger RNA which in turn came from DNA codes. Antibiotics like

Tetracycline interfere with this code interpretation step and prevent proteins from forming. That severely inhibits the life functions of bacteria because proteins are the executors of tasks coded by DNA. The result is the inability of bacteria to grow and multiply.

Viruses accomplish the same feat when they infect us. They hijack our ability to translate or read the DNA codes by tampering with our ribosome's assembly factory. They took over this ribosomal factory and stopped the manufacture of our own protein executives. By doing so, they effectively block the flow of information in the DNA operating system.

Viruses selectively use the host machinery to make copies of their viral executable codes for passing down their new offspring. It is like an army of 1,000 or 10,000 assuming control over millions of cells. Almost always, the number of soldiers in an army that invades a country will be vastly smaller than the total population of that country. Yet, the invading army succeeds in taking over territory because they would have first destroyed the central command, i.e. the king and his advisors. With no commands coming from the king, the subjects will accept orders from the aggressor.

Antibiotics like Penicillin attack the enemies by interfering with their cell wall synthesis. That makes the enemy bacteria weak and defenseless. Because the bacteria cell wall is like your skin, like the house for us and like a fortress for the kings.

How does the Penicillin antibiotic do this? Again, they do that by preventing information flow. A key material required in bacterial cell wall synthesis is called peptidoglycan, which is not possible to make from the DNA codes if Penicillin antibiotic is around. Like so many others, it is another information hacking tool.

The idea of information sabotage is not unique to microbes. That is, it is not a strategy only used by microbes against microbes. Plants use this strategy to defend against the microbes that infect them; they employ a novel information hacking strategy by generating molecules that prevent the viral and bacterial operating systems from functioning. The plant substances silence the RNA of the viruses. This means they prevent viruses from reading their coding program. The RNA executable code cannot be deciphered. This is because the plant substances block it. This strategy is called RNA silencing. It is a counter-defense strategy employed by plants. It is a tit-for-tat information war. If you attack by hacking, you get hit back by the same method.

RNA silencing is a useful tool in scientific research. Scientists adopt the RNA silencing method to investigate the functions of RNA coded in organisms. By silencing one RNA at a time, they deduce the functional role played by the information contained in that RNA and therefore the gene from which it was formed.

The truth is, we still do not know all the programs coded by each gene in our DNA Operating system. We have a good idea of the information content of many genes, but we have no ideas about many others. There are abundant program codes in the human DNA that do not constitute genes but possibly code for support functions in the cell. These program codes are interspersed within a gene—as well as in between genes.

For these DNA program codes to execute their function, they must first be translated into the language of RNA. This information is further used to create proteins. By knocking out RNA by using molecules obtained from plants or our own, we can guess their function. By absence, they make themselves conspicuously known.

Viruses can infect bacteria too. Viruses that infect bacteria are called Bacteriophages. So, viruses don't hit only multicellular life forms—they target unicellular life too. The amazing thing is even these unicellular life forms know how to protect themselves against cybercrime. The bacteria developed antivirus software that puts our computer anti-virus software to shame.

How do the bacteria defend themselves against this viral sabotage? They evolved an enzyme that cuts the viral executable codes! Like a saw used to cut timber, bacteria physically grab the viral RNA and shred them. This is like our office shredders used to get rid of unwanted information held in the form of paper.

Amazing stuff.

There are two medically relevant points related to bacteria-virus cyber warfare. Firstly, some scientists look at bacteriophages as potential anti-bacterial agents. They think bacteriophages could give us a means of fighting antibiotic-resistant bacteria.

If we run out of effective antibiotics, then what can we use to fight bacterial infections? The new antibiotic pipeline is drying up. This made scientists look for unconventional means and bacteriophages caught their attention for their ability to kill bacteria. Why don't we give patients a concoction of bacteriophages? There was a scientific paper published that described one such attempt. A patient in Alabama, US, was infected with a type of bacterium that was not responding to any available antibiotics. The patient became very ill and went into a coma for a few months. A team of doctors tried phage therapy. They gave this patient bacteriophages as medicine. The bacteria responsible for this patient's infection succumbed to the phages. The patient came out of his coma and got better.

The other medical angle of the bacteriophages story is their molecular saw that can cut DNA. This molecular saw, or molecular scissors, is an enzyme called Restriction Endonuclease. It is a mouthful of a name that can scare a layman. It is no exaggeration: this bacterial enzyme paved the way to a medical and scientific revolution called Genetic Engineering or Biotechnology. It transformed biology beyond recognition. For this reason, the discoverer of the Restriction endonuclease enzyme received apt recognition in the form of a Nobel Prize.

There is another exciting molecular biological tool possessed by bacteria and archaea for handling viral threats. This bacterial cyber technology uses a similar approach. The bacteria identify infecting viruses by means of characteristic gene sequences. This is like fingerprints or facial recognition used in criminology. When the viruses infect the bacteria, the bacteria scan virus gene sequences and copy part of it to keep in a gene database. These gene sequences are characteristically short and clustered and consist of palindromic repeats. For those who do not know about Palindromes, a Palindrome is a word that can be read forwards and backwards and still mean the same.

An example is the words level or civic. Read from front or back, they are the same.

Using stored viral recognition codes, when the same or related virus infects the bacteria again, a counterattack is unleashed that cuts and destroys the viral gene codes. The weapon used for this by the bacteria is an enzyme.

Palindromic gene sequences are often seen in the DNA of life systems. That is odd. Examples of palindromic gene codes are the ones used by the bacteria for recognition of gene codes of infecting viruses. CRISPR, short for Clustered Regularly Interspaced Short Palindromic Repeats is a microbial immune system that prokaryotes bacteria and archaea use to prevent infection using viruses called phages. At its core, the CRISPR system gives prokaryotes the ability to recognize precise genetic sequences matching a phage or other invaders and targeted these sequences for destruction using specialized enzymes.

The CRISPR bacterial defense system is now in the limelight because the 2020 Nobel Prize for Chemistry was awarded to two lady scientists who carried out pioneering research in this field. CRISPR bacterial cybertechnology is like the restriction endonuclease I referred to earlier.

Restriction endonuclease enzyme derived from the bacteria spurred a totally new scientific field called Biotechnology. CRISPR is said to be about 4 times more precise in the gene editing function and is a buzzword all over the world in all molecular biology laboratories. It is touted as the biggest advance in biological sciences since the discovery of DNA structure back in the 1950s.

CRISPR technology is poised to transform modern medicine by giving us the ability to correct and edit defective genes and cure genetic diseases. This technology also is being exploited to genetic modification of crops.

Restriction Endonuclease enzymes enables the Gene editing job and allows us to cut and paste portions of DNA information codes. It allows insertion of DNA codes any place desired. In short, it is the file editor we are familiar with in our computers. Until the advent of computers and the Microsoft Word application, we either wrote by hand or typed using the old-fashioned typewriters. Both these methods allowed little scope for editing. You cannot easily add new content between the typed lines. Microsoft Word changed everything. You can cut, delete and move words, sentences, paragraphs or even entire pages.

This is what Restriction Endonuclease enzymes did for us—gave a tool for gene editing. We can use this enzyme of bacterial origin (not a human invention) to insert genes, delete genes, and thereby alter gene programs.

Genetic engineering is like Aladdin's magical lamp giving us whatever we want. We use it for making customized medicines and foods. We acquired the ability to alter God's design. We are creating new things that did not exist in Nature. It is difficult to believe these tiny microbes made it all possible. I am not glorifying the science behind Genetic engineering.

My intention is to show how microbes gave us this technology.

The essence of Genetic engineering is simple. Bacteria assume the role of factories and make products we need. We attach the gene code for a medical product like, for example, insulin, to the bacterial DNA code. To do this, we pack the insulin gene code inside a viral carrier (bacteriophages with the natural ability to enter the bacterial interior) by using the Restriction endonuclease enzyme to cut the viral code and insert the insulin gene code. The virus goes inside and integrates its gene codes with the bacterial gene codes. When the bacteria start making their gene products, they inadvertently make the human insulin product too (which we sent through the viral courier). Then we extract the formed insulin product for our use. Until we discovered genetic engineering technology, we used primitive methods like extracting insulin by grinding up animal pancreas. Now we can instruct bacterial DNA programs to make a product of interest. We make protein medicines using this method which is heavily reliant on microbial technology. It is amazing that we take credit for it. It is common for us to do so. We take antibiotics from the microbial world and use it against them, don't we?

In the last couple of decades, we heard much about Genetically Modified foods (GM). It raised a lot of debate and fear among the public and politicians. The fear element was because these foods were grown using genetic technology and wondering what would happen if those new gene programs entered our bodies and started executing their codes.

I do not think the fear has subsided yet. In simple terms, what scientists did while modifying the gene codes of plants was insert special capacities in the plant programs they did not have before.

It could be a gene code for faster growth so that the crop can be harvested sooner. It could be a gene code with information necessary to fight plant pests to reduce the use of chemical pesticides. It could be a gene code for higher crop yields and so on. The necessary code instructions were inserted through code couriers—usually a microbe with the ability to infect plants. When they infect the plants, additional gene codes will get delivered. By the way, these scientists acted like hackers sending code instructions to the plants forcing them to comply.

Did you think of GM foods as the handiwork of legitimate gene hackers?

Man uses cut and paste gene editing technology to cure genetic diseases. Genetic diseases are due to faulty gene programs. It could be deletion of some gene codes, wrong programming codes or even insertion of unwanted codes. We use the restriction endonuclease enzyme to edit the faulty gene and thereby cure the hitherto incurable genetic diseases. Once again, we owe thanks to microbial technology.

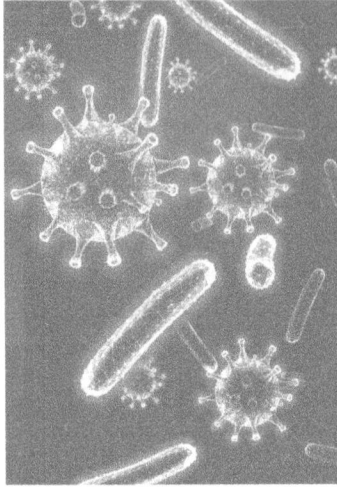

Chapter 14

THE GOOD SIDE OF MICROBES— EVERYDAY MICROBIAL BIOTECHNOLOGY IN OUR LIVES

THE DAILY TELEGRAPH newspaper from the UK published a story recently. Readers may remember the Chernobyl nuclear power plant disaster that happened in 1986. After this accident, the area was unfit for humans due to the high doses of background radiation from the nuclear spills.

Scientists studying this region found a microbe that can eat nuclear radiation to survive. How amazing. This is interesting for two reasons. One, the deadliest of our inventions (i.e., nuclear energy) is food for a microbe or two. Second, this microbe can help man to solve a problem that we cannot fix on our own. We dump millions of tons of nuclear waste. The UK alone is said to have 4.5 million cubic meters of nuclear waste we do not know what to do with. Is it possible that this microbe can be used to scavenge our nuclear mess?

Microbes are not new to scavenging. They scavenge dead

organisms of all sorts to return the atomic elements back to reusable form. Otherwise, the finite resources of atoms would forever get locked up in dead carcasses all over the planet. This throws open a new dimension to microbial existence. They are, after all, not here just to cause disease and death. They are not villains. At times, they may act the role of villains as a means of survival. The other side of microbes is that they can help, too. Scavenging is a useful function they can provide. In fact, it is an indispensable role that we cannot live without.

Microbes do other good things, too. They make it possible for life systems to generate the raw materials for making proteins, which means they basically enable the building blocks of life. I refer to a process called Nitrogen Fixation. Atmospheric Nitrogen is converted into ammonia which is then used for making amino acids, proteins, DNA and RNA.

These indispensable, vital molecules are all nitrogen-containing. If atmospheric Nitrogen could not be fixed to a form that can be used by us and other lifeforms, that's the end of the road for formation of life. Nitrogen Fixation is carried out naturally in soil by microorganisms, termed Diazotrophs, that include bacteria such as Azotobacter and Archaea. Some nitrogen-fixing bacteria have symbiotic relationships with leguminous plants.

It is not right to treat microorganisms with vengeance just because one of them caused the Corona crisis. I do not believe microbes exist for the sole purpose of disturbing our lives, not just our human lives, but also that of other life systems—especially when three-fourths of biomass is accounted for by microbes. I do not for a moment think Nature made all these diverse microbes just to create trouble. No system survives if they have no value. Nature would not have permitted a situation where the top-ranked, most populous creatures would be nothing but trouble. So, we need to learn to look at the positive side of these so-called crooked microbes.

Wherever possible, life systems on Earth adopt a cooperative approach. It is not always possible when there are too many systems out there. Even within human society, the

Homo sapiens species is divided into too many factions based on geography, religion and skin color.

We have yet to see a conflict-free approach to living and that being the case within a species, it is too much to ask for blissful peace between organisms. Yet, there is still a lot of cooperation and tolerance between life systems. The practice of agriculture and gardening adopted by Homo sapiens is reflective of a symbiotic relationship between man and a variety of plant species where there is mutual benefit.

Domestication of animals is another area where man and animals live in peace. The question is: what sort of relationship do we enjoy between man and microbes? I cannot accept the theory that microbes are waiting for a chance to cause disease and death in man and other lifeforms.

Let us start first by exploring the possible applications of the viruses which are, as I said before, the most predominant life form on Earth. It is estimated that the oceans have as many as 1,028 forms of bacteria.

That is a lot of bacteria.

Water, therefore, is a broth of bacteria and one could safely suspect it is not safe to mess with water. Would you be happy to live in unsafe conditions where all that indispensable water is actually a carrier for microbes like bacteria to gain access to animal hosts? What happens in Nature is interesting.

There are viruses in the same ocean water, probably in equivalent amounts to bacteria, which can infect the bacteria. The viruses that infect bacteria are called Bacteriophages. Bacteriophages are present in rivers and ocean water in great numbers. Every milliliter of water contains 100 million bacteriophages.

We used to watch news channels with bated breath to hear the latest Corona case statistics. Most people's hearts skipped beat when they read the news that so many new cases were identified and that so many people died. On average, daily, about 250,000 more people were infected by the Corona virus worldwide and about 5,000-7,000 people died every day. You begin to wonder when it will be your turn to become part of those statistics.

Do you have any idea of the rate at which the bacteriophage viruses in water infect the bacteria? Every second (yes, every second) about 10^{23} viruses infect the bacteria in water bodies.

Again, you must be as proficient in mathematics as Ramanujam to comprehend the numbers. Don't be fooled by the expression of the number as 10^{23} because it is 10 multiplied by 10 a total of 23 times. This will run into quadrillions.

At this rate of attack, the bacteriophages kill 20-40% of world's bacteria in water bodies daily. Do you see, as I see, a possible benefit for the existence of viruses? But for the check imposed by bacteriophages, it is possible that bacteria in water bodies could grow exponentially to the point the water could become unusable for life systems because water becomes more concentrated with bacteria making it more toxic.

Or the bacteria could use up the raw materials for making more bacterial offspring at such a pace that there would soon be a shortage of elements for use by other lifeforms. Bacteria would use them all up and there would be nothing left for others. The bacterial reproductive multiplication time is just 20 minutes. Every 20 minutes, the next generation of bacteria is born. So, you can easily imagine the explosive increase in population of bacteria if left unchecked.

One of the biggest concerns we have is the exploding human population and how the Earth will support the rising population. There are people who already believe that our current population of 7.8 billion is way above the limit of sustainability. This is just for one species. What about other life forms? Do you see my point? We cannot leave everything for the bacteria to use, can we?

People do not hesitate to go to the doctor when they feel unwell. Quite often the cause of their illness is the invasion of our body by a microbe and the impending or ongoing man-microbe war. This will usually be evident by the fever, cough and symptoms like that. Fever is an alarm bell sounded by the body when a microbial war threat is perceived. It is like a war siren.

Fever is a natural body response to kill the microbe,

possibly a virus, with body heat. It is a protective response. But what do we do? We take Paracetamol to lower the fever, which interferes with the body's strategy to fight the microbe.

Viruses generally do not tolerate heat. They prefer cold climates. That is why they strike in the winter. They lurk in cold beverages, ice cream, etc. Once you consume them, the viruses sneak in. Socially, we have the habit of drinking hot cups of tea or soup, which we do more often when we have a common cold. In fact, this is our body's signal to send in hot beverages to kill the virus hiding in the throat.

In the winter, we don't prefer cold drinks because we don't feel like drinking a cold drink when the outside temperature is freezing. The same cold drink will be welcomed in hot climates. Our body helps us indirectly by altering our taste preferences based on the seasons.

Heat kills microbes. That is why it is recommended that drinking water should be boiled and filtered before drinking. In less developed countries, clean water is not readily available in all places. People drink water from unclean sources. WHO recommends boiling the water before drinking and this makes it possible for a significant amount of world population to get potable water.

Deadly gut pathogens—including the Cholera bacteria—succumb to our heat. We use thermal energy to disrupt and damage the DNA or RNA codes and proteins of these pathogens. That is what boiling is all about. These macromolecules in life systems cannot tolerate temperatures of 100 degrees centigrade. Proteins get denatured and DNA molecules are sheared apart. We know boiling kills the pathogens, but we hardly know the biotechnology behind it.

Our dishwashers and washing machines can now operate at high temperatures of 80-100 degrees centigrade. They were designed purposely for killing the microbes likely to hide in utensils or clothes. Steam-based dry-cleaning works on the same principle. Hospitals use autoclaves for sterilization of medical equipment so that they can be re-used on patients. This is a very important part of the infection control practices of a hospital.

The basis of this technology is heat-induced disruption of microbial structures to kill them.

In rural India, and I suppose many other parts of the world, having a refrigerator at home is a luxury not available in all homes. This was at least the case in India not long ago. What do people do when they have milk or curry left over from the day? They heat it up before going to sleep. They may be illiterate and may not know why they are doing it. All they know is that heating the leftover food prolongs the time it takes to deteriorate. They are applying thermal energy to kill the microbes that entered the food through air or water. Microbes are everywhere. Always, they are present all around in the air you breathe. They settle on everything, everywhere.

Nowadays, the worldwide standard practice is to store our food in refrigerators. We store many items—like meat—in freezers. By doing so, we turn into biochemists. We employ the principle of heat kinetics to modulate the action of enzymes. Biochemists would tell you that if you plotted a graph with temperature on one axis and the rate of an enzyme action on the other, then you will find that the action of enzyme increases as the temperature increases.

However, this cannot go on forever. When temperatures increase beyond 70 or 80 degrees centigrade, the thermal energy becomes strong enough to disrupt the orderly arrangement of biomolecules such as enzymes. They will be broken apart. The molecules will be ripped apart by the force of heat energy. If the temperature drops to below 15 degrees centigrade, then biochemical enzymes will slow down and run like slow motion. Life itself becomes a slow-motion film.

The optimum temperature for biological enzymes to work is around 35-37 degrees centigrade—which happens to be the normal body temperature. Our body and its metabolism evolved to maintain the temperatures needed for our metabolic enzymes to work optimally. If your body temperature is cooled to below 20 or 25 degrees centigrade, your metabolism slows down. When you cool below that temperature, hypothermia sets in and body enzymes start shutting down. So hypothermia is all about biochemically shutting down the body production factory. We evolved, like many other creatures, to be warm-blooded animals, meaning that we maintain our body temperature to within a few degrees of fluctuation irrespective of the outside temperature. But freezing water and ice can overcome the body's homeostatic ability, i.e., the ability to keep constant the internal body environment.

Science fiction films talk about freezing astronauts during space travel so their body metabolism can be nearly shut down, reducing their energy needs during the long space travel. This is the same principle as keeping your meat in freezers, unspoiled for months. Polar bears implement this method by hibernating for six months in winter when the food supply in the icy climate is scarce. They drastically reduce their energy needs because all their body enzymes are literally stopped.

The idea of storing our food in freezers is that the microbes cannot function at that low temperature and therefore the degradation of food by microbial enzymes does not happen. In other words, degradation of food, which we call spoilage, is due to microbes that settle on their surface from the air and water all around us. It is said that 30-40% of food grown worldwide is wasted. This is due to procurement beyond needs or simply careless storage.

But it is the microbes that return the atomic elements locked in these foods back into circulation by attacking all bio-matter, leftover food or dead bodies. They extract food energy in the process of this ever-useful recycling of matter and so they also get to live. It is a dual-purpose exercise. But for this atomic recycling, all matter would forever be locked up in dead carcasses or wasted food. Please remember they are not making new atoms on our planet. Atoms, in fact, were never made on earth. What we got is what we got. They came from distant stars in finite quantities. The job of a life system is to juggle these atoms and keep up the game of life.

We preserve dead bodies on ice awaiting funeral arrangements. Again, this is a biochemical effort to dampen the kinetics of microbial enzymes and slow the body's decay. When someone dies, the microbes inside and outside the body attack it like hyenas attack a carcass. This is a biochemical attack launched by the microbial enzymes on the dead body because the dead body is full of biochemical molecules. The microbes generate energy for their survival. Some waste products are released, which are usually gaseous. Carbon dioxide and methane gases are produced along with some acids. If the dead body was sunk in deep waters, it would rise to the surface of the water, buoyed by the microbial gas waste. That is bad news for a cunning killer who thought he could get away with a heinous crime.

I need to mention here a unique life system that defies the heat energy and in fact preferentially survives in hot springs. It is a microbe called Thermus aquaticus. It lives in natural hot environments where the temperature can be as high as 80 degrees centigrade. Why is this important? Because this bacterium and its heat-resistant technology paved the way for one of the biggest scientific developments called the Polymerase Chain Reaction (PCR). It would be no exaggeration if I said this PCR technique turned the field of science and medicine upside down. It has had an impact that is too difficult to quantify.

Basically, the PCR technique involves copying a DNA code and making lots of them. The idea is to sequentially use the copies to make further copies. In life systems, that is what happens during cell division. DNA code is copied by the enzyme DNA polymerase to be passed on to the daughter cell. To make a copy, the DNA polymerase enzyme must first bind to the DNA code sequence and read it like a bar code. After reading the DNA, the polymerase enzyme separates and falls away.

Kary Mullis, the biochemist who discovered PCR technology, was working on a project where he had to make copies of some DNA codes. He imagined how nice it would be if this could be automated so that the same DNA polymerase could be used to continuously make copies of a given DNA code.

For this, the DNA polymerase should be allowed to anneal (combine) with a given DNA code to be copied. After copying, the DNA polymerase enzyme detaches so it can be ready to make another copy of the same DNA code. It was already known that cooling allowed the DNA polymerase to combine with a DNA code—while heating separates it. The temperature needed to separate the enzyme and the DNA code is above 80 degrees centigrade. However, this heat would also destroy the DNA polymerase enzyme. If the enzyme was stable enough to withstand this high temperature, then the DNA polymerase enzyme could be cyclically used to first combine with a given DNA code and separate from it and repeat the cycle endlessly.

The result is an exponential increase in the number of DNA copies. This allows scientists and doctors to have enough of the DNA material to study them. Since life systems use such miniscule quantities of the DNA codes, it is not possible to extract enough of it to study them meaningfully. PCR technology enabled making abundant copies of the DNA code present in miniscule quantities. The PCR process is very useful in science and medicine. Even diagnosis of Corona virus is done by the same PCR technology.

The problem faced by Kary Mullis was how to automate the assembly and disassembly of the DNA polymerase enzyme with the DNA code it copies. For that he needed a DNA polymerase enzyme that can withstand temperatures above 80 degrees centigrade. In conventional life systems, no enzyme or protein can withstand such harsh temperatures.

Fortunately, in the early 1960s, a group of researchers found a microbe living in the Yellowstone Mushroom spring (Thermas aquaticus) which preferentially lives in this hot environment. This microbe adapted to the extreme hot conditions and found an evolutionary solution to maintain the integrity of the proteins and enzymes at temperatures above 80 degrees centigrade.

Kary Mullis said in his book, *Dancing Naked in the Mind Field*, that one fine day as he was driving back from work, he had the heavenly insight of using this heat-resistant form of DNA polymerase for repetitive DNA copying cycles. This enzyme is the Taq polymerase (Taq = Thermus aquaticus).

This long story illustrates two things. Microbes have unique capabilities such as extreme heat resistance which not many life systems on earth can boast of. Perhaps you would find such life systems on an alien planet where the normal temperatures are very high.

The second and more important point is that microbes are sources of amazing technologies we can commercially exploit. PCR technology is one. I mentioned before that the medical miracle of antibiotics is a product of microbes. Nitrogen fixation, the root source of proteins for all life systems on earth, is a bacterial technology. There is a bacterium identified in the Chernobyl nuclear facility site that can eat and clear nuclear waste which is being looked on as a savior. There are bacteria that can eat and clean oil spills. The list goes on and on.

Microbes are central to the art of preparing bio-fertilizers. These days, people are becoming more conscious of organically grown foods because they are afraid of the unhealthy chemicals used as fertilizers and pesticides. There is a tendency across the world to reduce the use of chemical agents in agriculture. In many parts of the world, even illiterate farmers now turn to generation of bio-fertilizers.

Phosphate and Nitrogen are essential nutrients for plants. Phosphate is abundant in the soil but remains mostly bound to other soil components. Nitrogen is abundant in the air. A fungus called Penicillium billai can unlock the phosphate locked up in the soil—making it accessible to plant roots. It achieves this feat by making an organic acid which dissolves the phosphates in the soil. Bio-fertilizer is made by coating this fungus on seeds and planting them or by directly placing them in the ground around plant roots. The friendly fungus will wrap around the roots and, apart from phosphate hunting, can also help in preventing the growth of other dangerous organisms near the root and thereby avoid plant diseases.

Rhizobium is another example of a bio-fertilizer. They live in the plant roots in what are called nodules. These nodules are biological factories absorbing nitrogen from the atmospheric air and converting it into an organic form that can be assimilated by plants. This is called Nitrogen fixation, as I said earlier. Rhizobium occurs in nature as such and is a natural fertilizer made by God.

It is common in rural parts of the world where farmers collect all biological wastes like rotting leaves, decaying food, and degradable biological matter and composting them. By doing so they can convert decomposed organic matter into a humus called compost, which is good fertilizer for plants. The architect of this composting process is the microbe. They cause the biochemical disassembly of organic molecules—liberating the essential nutrients back to the soil for the use of plants.

In short, microbes are key players in the global management of atomic matter. This is no different from recycling plastic, glass bottles, paper, metals, etc. Microbes are the ultimate recyclers.

Continuing with the topic of biotechnology in action, let us look at a process called Fermentation. This is the process that gives us bread, cakes, doughnuts, croissants, yoghurt, cultured milk products like Kefir (made by adding yeast and bacteria to milk) and alcoholic beverages. Tempeh and Miso are products made from fermented soya beans. A South Indian food item called Idly is made by fermenting rice and lentils overnight and grinding them into a batter that can be steam cooked. Kimchi is a popular Korean dish made from fermented cabbage.

Basically, fermentation means extracting energy from carbohydrates in the absence of oxygen. The key player in this controlled process is the microbe. Carbohydrate-rich food is allowed acted on by a microbe such as yeast, which extracts energy from food for its own use and leaves behind waste products. These waste products are of use to us and that is why we deliberately make this process happen. Since the Neolithic age, humans used fermentation to make beverages and foods.

During the fermentation process, beneficial microbes like yeast, molds and bacteria break down sugars and starches into alcohols and acids, making food more nutritious and preserving it so people can store it for longer periods of time without it spoiling.

Fermentation also aids in pre-digestion. During the fermentation process, microbes feed on sugars and starches, breaking down food before anyone has even consumed it. This is the reason why people ferment some types of foods.

There are three basic forms of fermentation. Lactic acid fermentation is when yeasts and bacteria convert starches or sugars into lactic acid in foods like sauerkraut, kimchi, pickles, yoghurt and sourdough bread. Ethyl alcohol fermentation is where pyruvate molecules in starches or sugars are broken down by yeasts into alcohol and carbon dioxide molecules to produce wine and beer. Acetic acid fermentation of starches or sugars from grains or fruit converts them into sour tasting vinegar and condiments. Each of these kinds of fermentation is due to the work of microbes specialized at converting certain substances into others.

Can you comprehend the extent that microbes play a role in human living? Without them we do not have alcohol and wines and the whole big industry would vanish. You would not have pubs or bars. What would human life be without them?

Imagine a world without cakes, bread, buns and biscuits. Microbes like yeast are responsible for your bakeries. Yeast converts sugar to carbon dioxide and alcohol in the absence of oxygen, causing dough to rise. But for the biotechnology of the yeasts, you would not be having your birthday cakes and wedding cakes. What kind of a lousy world would that be? Man's staple diet of bread would be non-existent if yeasts did not act on our dough. We would be eating the grains instead.

Without microbes, we would not have condiments in our diet.

Our own gut is a place where a lot of fermentation happens inside us caused by the action of the microbes that live there. As mentioned earlier, fermentation is metabolism in the absence of oxygen. The lower gut is largely devoid of oxygen and becomes a perfect place for microbial fermentation reactions. Products of these microbial fermentation reactions have nutritious value. They also help modulate our immunity.

Elevated concentrations of mostly acidic fermentation by-products create an inhospitable environment for the dangerous bacteria that come into the gut. Thereby, intestinal microbes do the same job as food preservatives where the production of acids makes it difficult for other microbes to settle in and spoil the food. Our lives are full of surprises like this, where unknowingly we indulge in bio-warfare. You never thought of condiment making as something involving an ecological competition between microbes, did you?

Certain exogenous, plant-derived polyphenols can be bio-transformed to compounds with antioxidant, anti-cancer and or anti-inflammatory properties by gut microbes which improve their absorption by our gut. Microbes offer a pharmaceutical service for us.

To sum up, the world of microbes is full of good things. Unfortunately, few people are aware of this—we think of microbes as creatures to be hated.

The Corona virus pandemic accentuated this belief beyond repair.

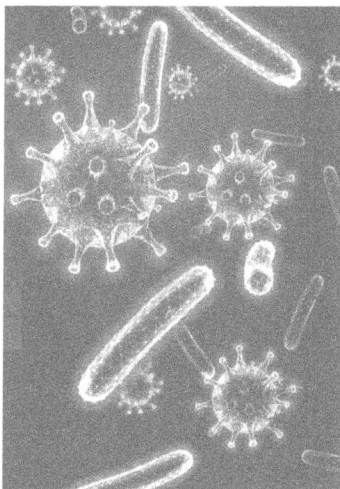

Chapter 15

EXPLOITING NATURE FOR ANTI-MICROBIAL WARFARE TECHNOLOGY

MICROBES HAVE EXISTED on earth for a long time. I alluded to the man-microbe relations in some detail already. Microbes build relationships with other lifeforms too. The relationships may not always be cordial. Microbes often show their evil faces. It is true there are many cases where microbes co-evolved symbiotic relationships with higher life forms.

As I said before, there is a degree of mistrust between life systems. Both parties are to be blamed. Because of the lack of trust, the life systems have evolved various strategies to combat the perceived threat.

The only good thing about these wars is that they are fought between different types of life systems. The enemy is a member of an unrelated species. These wars are unlike the wars we human fight. We are used to fighting between us, which other life systems never do. That is a unique feature of humanity.

Enormous resources are wasted by man for fighting man. As a life system, we also have combat strategies to fight the microbes. Our immune systems are well-equipped armies that help us in this combat, but microbes evolved evasive strategies to overcome these attacks.

One thing unique about man is his ability to borrow technology from other lifeforms using so-called scientific methods. Antibiotics used in modern medicine are products obtained from Nature and not man-made. Of course, we make them in pharmaceutical factories that enrich corporations. But the idea was not original.

Between 1981 and 2001, there were 109 new antibiotics that came into use world-wide. To bring a new medicine into the market these days, pharmaceutical companies conduct extensive clinical trials taking years. There are drug regulatory agencies in each country evaluating these applications and if found safe and effective, they will be licensed for human use.

USA has the Food and Drug Administration (FDA) and Europe has the European Medicines Agency (EMA). There are other national regulatory bodies in Europe. Of the 109 antibiotics that came into human use, 90% of them were derived from natural sources. With this kind of information, the talk about advances in medicine comes under question.

We learned about the existence of microbes only within the last couple of centuries, after the discovery of microscopes in the 17th century by Robert Hooke and Antony Von Leeuwenhoek.

But microbes were around for a long time before that. They went about their lives and while we minded our own. Microbes do what microbes do. They have been infecting man just like they infect other lifeforms. Without knowing the origins of these infections, we had traditional ways of treating them.

Egyptians and the Greeks knew some molds and plant extracts were effective treatments for infections. This was wisdom passed down from their ancestors. They had no idea about the root cause of their infections and had no idea why molds and plants helped to cure infections. Knowledge gained by empirical use of these natural recipes helped them and no one cared how they worked.

Even today we have various forms of alternate medical practices like Ayurveda, Unani, Siddha and Acupuncture employing natural products to heal various forms of diseases. These treatments really work. The World Health Organization (WHO) endorsed the continued use of these ancient medical practices as useful for humanity.

Today we do not hesitate to go to the doctor for minor ailments. We do not hesitate to even self-prescribe an antibiotic if we have throat infections. We use antibiotics and antiseptic creams on our wounds. Our forefathers who lived as recently as early 20th century did not have these luxuries. They died in clusters due to infections. They were sitting ducks in the eyes of the microbes. They were defenseless. My great grandfather apparently died of a tooth infection. How many of us these days die of a simple tooth infection? Soldiers who fought in the wars died of infections of their wounds rather than the wounds themselves.

Our war against microbes intensified in the last 70 years since the chance discovery of Penicillin antibiotic by Alexander Fleming in 1928. Fleming had the hobby of growing microbes in jars. He had such bacterial broths on his worktable. It took another 14 years for 3 other researchers to find out the killer substance was the antibiotic called Penicillin made by the mold Penicillium Chrysogenum.

In 1952 another researcher called Selman Waksman received a Nobel Prize for the discovery of Streptomycin antibiotic used for the treatment of TB. He isolated this antibiotic from another mold called Streptomyces. He was able to make this discovery by collecting soil and water samples from different locations and studying the microbes living in those environments.

Over the next 20 years, pharmaceutical companies followed the same strategy of collecting and analyzing soil and water samples from all over the world. This led to the discovery of many new antibiotics. The diversity and density of microbes living in natural environments is unbelievable.

For example, a spoonful of soil from the Amazonian rainforest is estimated to contain about 1,800 types of microbes. One can only imagine what each of those microbes can do. It is a moot point. What are the losses we potentially face from purely a medical standpoint by deforestation of rainforests like the Amazon?

We could lose any number of valuable medicines before we even know about them. What a sad loss. It is like writing amazing books and destroying them before anyone can read them. Ignorance of a large section of our public leads to the loss of invaluable medicinal compounds plants and microbes were ready to give us.

Plants are veritable sources of antimicrobial substances. They make them for two reasons. The first is to protect themselves from microbes and pests which is a motif that is biologically licensed. It is the right of every life system to protect itself by hook or crook. This is Darwin's principle of the survival of the fittest.

The second reason why plants make medically relevant substances is for the benefit of other life systems like us. For example, the Cinchona tree makes the antimalarial drug called Quinine. Why would a tree make the antimalarial drug if the malaria parasite does not even bother it? Do you see what I mean?

A tree called Artemisa annua makes another antimalarial drug called Artemisinin. Discovery of Artemisinin led to the award of a Nobel Prize to the Chinese scientist involved. The deserving candidate for this Nobel Prize is the tree Artemisa. I know it sounds absurd, but some readers will understand what I am saying. Plants are much better organic chemists than us.

The ancient Chinese knew about the medical benefits of Artemisa plant for the treatment of intermittent fever. Intermittent fever is a characteristic hallmark of Malarial infection. The Chinese did not know the causative agent of the Malaria infection, but they did know of a medicinal product obtained from the Artemisa tree. This illustrates the possibility that many so-called quack remedies of Chinese medicine may be based on something real.

Medicines found in nature (made by plants or microbes) are like raw grains or fruits that we grow in fields. These grains and fruits are processed by our factories to create the hundreds of food items we buy in the supermarket. Food industries package them in nice, flashy, attractive packs bearing no resemblance to the raw grains or fruits that went into them.

The Kellogg cereal you eat looks a lot different from the raw material that went into its production. The chocolate you ate from the colorful pack is cocoa beans and sugar from a sugarcane plant. We also see a lot of different company names that claim to have manufactured these foods though the real manufacturer was the plant that grew on its own.

In the same way medically active substances made by plants or microbes are modified and packed in the form of tablets, capsules or injections by the pharmaceutical companies while the real pharmacist was the plant that grew in the forest or the soil microbe. But we have doctors who trained from top medical schools prescribing them for us while they are doing the same job as the natural village healer who never went to any school.

If plants and soil microbes did not make pharmacologically active molecules, our drug formularies would be small and grossly inadequate to treat all sorts of diseases that we suffer. This is a fact that nobody can refute. Plants and microbes are our real pharmaceutical research and development corporations. What the real pharmaceutical companies do is just a bit of tinkering here and there to make improvements.

Finding a drug made by our pharmaceutical companies from scratch is a rarity. They prefer not to re-invent the wheel. More importantly, they do not pay a fortune in royalties to the microbe and there will never be an intellectual property dispute.

That is the real attraction.

Now we go to the next question. Why do plants make medicinal substances? I claim that they make it to benefit us just like they give us fruits and vegetables for food. I feel the food and medicines are the contributions made by the plants in the symbiotic relationship between man and plants. What do we give the plants back? We look after them by providing nutrients and water. We call it agriculture. Both parties won.

We use several antimicrobials in our daily life. We started using them more after the Corona virus scare. In rural parts of India, villagers have the custom of applying a dilute paste of cow dung in and around the house. This is a regular occurrence in the houses of the village. Scientific studies have shown that extracts of cow dung have antibacterial activity against pathogens like E. coli, Pseudomonas and S. aureus. It was also effective against the fungus Candida, as well. Cow dung was and is the sanitizer in rural India.

There are many herbs known to different geographically distinct populations. It happens that the medicines derived from these herbs are specific and relevant for those local geographies. Often people use these herbs as a Nutraceutical which literally means something that has value both as a pharmacological substance and a food item.

Cinnamon, for example, has antimicrobial and antioxidant properties and is widely used as a food item in many parts of the world. Turmeric is a household cooking ingredient in India. It has significant antimicrobial properties. The active constituent of Turmeric is said to be the Curcumin molecule which provides these medicinal benefits.

There are so many other herbs like Tulsi (Basil), Garlic, Pepper, Ginger, Lime, etc. that have medicinal values. Eugenol, an oily compound present in clove, cinnamon, ginger, star anise, galangal, basil, bay leaf and nutmeg, is used as an antiseptic though we only know of these culinary additives for their flavor. It is used by dentists for antiseptic and anti-inflammatory properties. They often apply it on the gums to kill germs and relieve the pain of dental procedures.

Eugenol is a common ingredient in toothpaste, mouthwashes, soaps, insect repellants, perfumes, etc. It looks like a lot of our activities of modern clean living need the handiwork of plants to keep the microbes away. Studies show that Eugenol is almost twice as effective as the antifungal drug Nystatin in killing Candida. Eugenol, or oil of clove, is used in some countries to treat fungal infections of the skin, ear and genitals.

Neem trees contain about 140 active compounds with medicinal properties—including antimicrobial. Neem trees produce compounds that can kill viruses, bacteria (including TB and Cholera) and even the Malaria pathogen. Products made from the Neem tree have been used for medicinal purposes for over two millennia in India.

Neem trees generate molecular compounds by organic chemical synthesis with anti-parasitic, antifungal, antibacterial and antiviral properties. Nimbidin is the main antibacterial agent present in the Neem tree. Together with a similar compound called Nimbinin, it has an additional anti-insecticidal property. In India farmers use Neem-coated urea as a fertilizer that helps them avoid pesticides. There was a claim that Neem is useful in COVID-19 treatment which was not scientifically proven but there is empirical evidence it might be effective against the Corona virus.

In India it is a traditional practice to tie a bunch of Neem leaves at the doorstep of a house where someone had smallpox or chickenpox. It is said to notify the residents of the village to keep away and maintain social distancing. At the same time, Neem is thought to purify the air with its antiviral properties.

Neem trees produce biochemical compounds for their own protection. Like other plants, the Neem tree is susceptible to fungal and bacterial diseases. The medicinal substances I mentioned are products evolved by the Neem tree for its personal combat with the microbes that threaten its existence.

Incidentally, we use them for our protection as well. Just like we use antibiotics (made by the microbes to kill their competitors) made by natural sources we also use the Neem tree and a variety of other plant-based products with antimicrobial properties.

A tricky question arises when we look at the anti-cancer properties of the plant products. Plants are not known to get cancers like we do. Some excessive multiplication of plant cells does happen, which may look like a plant tumor, but this is usually caused by bacterium, virus or fungus. So, they are not genetic code alterations like what happens in human cancers. The other thing about the plant tumors is they never spread (metastasize like our human tumors).

In short, one could say plants do not get cancer like us and do not die of cancer. The bacterium Agrobacterium tumefaciens is one of the most common culprits in plant tumor origin and is the cause of the crown gall. Fungal infection like black knot, caused by Dibotryon morbosum, is another common plant tumor. My question is, why do the plants make anti-cancer molecules if they do not suffer from human-like cancer?

Plants make a lot of anticancer molecules. Vincristine and Vinblastine were isolated from the Madagascar periwinkle plant in the 1950s. These molecules act by interfering with the cell division of the cancer cells and are used for the treatment of several types of cancers.

The mistletoe plant has anticancer molecules called viscotoxins. Taxanes are another class of anticancer drugs isolated from the Pacific Yew tree. They are mitosis inhibitors. These drugs are widely used in modern medicine. I do not want to list all types of anticancer molecules found in plants because, if I did, it would bore readers. Suffice to say that there are as many as 12 different classes of cancer medicines found in plants and my question is, for what?

I am inclined to believe these molecules are created for the benefit of man. The concept is not difficult to grasp if one thinks about the source of all our food. Why should plants make our food? Just like the food industry is a multi-billion-dollar business, the Oncology drug market is also highly lucrative.

Plants are good business partners to mankind, and they seem to be the bigger contributors to the collaboration. In many cases plants seem to be selflessly working for our benefit.

A common theme in the mechanism of action of the plant-derived cancer agents is the inhibition of mitosis, the cell division. Biology students know that mitosis, the process by which the cell divides into two, involves a spindle made of protein molecules called tubulin. Tubulin proteins are laid like we lay tracks for moving goods. The newly formed cells are moved on these tubulin tracks. Plant-derived cancer agents work so these tubulin tracks cannot be laid for moving the goods used in the cell division process.

It surprises me that some marine lifeforms make anticancer drugs, God knows why. An anti-cancer drug called Psammaplin is made by marine microalgae, cyanobacteria and heterotrophic bacteria living in association with invertebrates like sponges, corals and tunicates. This agent prevents tumor cell invasion and new blood vessel formation within the tumors, thereby attacking cancers. Didemnin is a peptide anticancer drug isolated from a marine tunicate which inhibits a variety of tumors.

I can list a few more anticancer drugs found in marine life, but I'll stop here. I want to ask the same questions I raised for the plants.

Why would marine life forms make these anticancer agents? Why do plants give us food? Why does marine life, like fish, give food?

If plants and marine life are designed to give us food, then what stops them from going one step farther to give us medicines?

We should view these designs in nature as a form of symbiotic relationships between life systems. Nature allows co-evolution of various life systems such that there is a build-up of mutually beneficial relationships.

On that basis, I propose that disease-causing pathogenic microbes (like the Corona virus) are Nature's cybernetic control of the rising population—which has become unsustainable.

At the risk of severe criticism, I assert that microbial pathogens have a role to play in keeping our population in check.

That is their biological role.

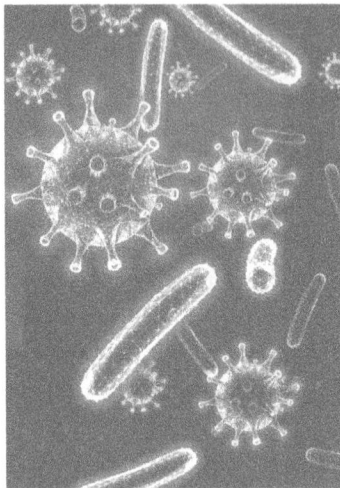

Chapter 16

OXYGEN COMBUSTION: TECHNOLOGY TRANSFER BETWEEN MICROBES

IF ONE EXAMINES man-microbe relations in minute detail and count how many microbes are good for us (by performing essential metabolic or protective roles in return for favors from us), bad to us (by causing disease and death) and neutral to us (do not affect us but focus their attention on other lifeforms) we would get a nice picture.

It is likely that our immune system evolved towards aggression towards bad microbes and ignoring the biological design or reason behind it.

I find this very difficult to grasp.

I bring to your attention the fact our doctors often curb immune response by using anti-inflammatory and immunosuppressant drugs. By doing so, they interfere with Nature's design, but the outcome of their intervention is beneficial from a medical standpoint because, in many cases, the damage caused by our immune attack is more severe than the disease itself.

I suppose we as a life system try selfish evolutionary strategies to preserve our species—which is okay in the biological world. All lifeforms were given the freedom to self-preserve. But there is something over and above the selfish motifs that someone or something (God?) must take care of.

This is the Greater Good.

In a religious sense, Hindu philosophy calls it Dharma. While individual living species may be hell-bent to preserve themselves (such as fighting death-causing microbes) the planet behaves like a Complex System which manifests self-regulatory properties that limits excesses. For the Complex System (in this case the Earth) it is not personal. It has no obligation to defend humanity or protect people over and above other lifeforms. Earth as a Complex System exhibits benevolent features that result in a lot of good.

Cyanobacteria, also known as blue-green algae, helped produce oxygen on the planet by conducting photosynthesis. That is the biological job for which they evolved. By doing so, these microbes caused a paradigm shift in the way energy generation happened in life systems. Their contribution led to the formation of oxygen almost 2.7 billion years ago. Earth was devoid of oxygen until then and all life forms that existed before that relied on energy sources that did not require combustion in the presence of oxygen.

They were anaerobic and could not make large quantities of energy which led to the limitation on the size of the life form. They essentially remained single-celled. Appearance of oxygen, thanks to the microbe called cyanobacteria, made it possible for lifeforms to use oxygen to combust their energy fuels and generate more energy.

This helped life forms grow bigger and become multicellular. In short, a tiny microbe made all the difference in the growth and evolution of multicellular life. This is like the discovery of oil that transformed transportation and industry. Oil to our industry is like oxygen to life systems. That makes the contribution of microbes in this epoch-making contribution more important.

Before we move on, I want to highlight another earth-shattering advance in life systems made possible by the microbes. All life forms that existed on earth before the advent of oxygen were unicellular and anaerobic. They did not know how to deal with oxygen when it appeared on the planet.

In fact, these early life forms found oxygen very toxic. They perished due to oxygen, which is unbelievable considering that life forms only die now due to lack of oxygen and not because of oxygen. Over time, there appeared one or two microbes that evolved the capacity to handle oxygen. In fact, they found a way to tame the oxygen's fury and make it work for life systems. This is like the combustion engine technology that came about a couple of centuries ago. Combustion engine technology helped to burn the fuel with oxygen and the amount of energy released was much more than before. This is the difference between horsepower and motor-power.

For a long time, there existed on earth two types of lifeforms. One type was capable of living with oxygen. Another form of life existed which could not handle oxygen. The life forms that could handle oxygen became energy-rich. The amount of power they could generate proved to be more than enough for a single-celled organism. They became capable of supporting a union of many cells. This was the origin of multicellular life.

If you had valuable technology, what would you do? Normally people sell the technology to others who may need it. This is all about commerce and cooperation. This is what happened in the early earth. The unicellular life form that had the oxygen-combusting technology entered into a collaboration with the organism that did not have this technology.

This was like the union of the horse-drawn carriage design with oxygen-combusting engine. It is said that Henry Ford faced the same situation when pioneering car design, and he found a way to make a petrol-combusting engine to drive the car.

Early life forms had the same need.

What eventually happened was oxygen-busting bacteria agreed to a symbiotic relation whereby it enters the cell of an anaerobic lifeform and stays inside.

In other words, the anaerobic life form agrees to accommodate the oxygen-busting bacteria in its home with the promise that this tenant will provide a contribution in the form of oxygen-driven energy capture. It is alleged, with valid evidence, that this tenant bacteria evolved into the mitochondria that populates every cell. These mitochondria are independent lifeforms living in perfect harmony with another lifeform and one cannot find another example of a perfect marriage.

Energy was the prize life systems were after. It was like the gold rush. All life forms need energy to run their processes. Plants were unlike animals because they could not physically move around and hunt their food down. They found another way of capturing energy. They focused on a source of energy that was endless and probably will not run out for a few more billion years. It is photosynthesis I am talking about.

Plant cells have Chloroplasts which are subcellular organelles involved with tapping the sun's energy. This process is called Photosynthesis. They use the light-sensitive pigments called Chlorophyll to absorb sunlight energy and convert it into electrical energy. The energy of the sunlight is used to knock off electrons and conduct them, or let them flow, which is literally electricity. The principle behind this is the Photoelectric effect which Einstein elucidated back in 1910. He was awarded the Nobel Prize for this discovery and not for the Relativity Theory as many believe.

Another point worth noting is that solar panels used for solar power generation work on the same principle as how plant leaves work. Every plant leaf is a solar panel.

Why are we suddenly talking of plants, photosynthesis and solar panels? What relevance do they have to the topic of microbes? Yes, it is relevant.

Once upon a time, the so-called Chloroplast was a free-living microbe. Now it lives in a permanent symbiotic relation with plants by residing inside the plant cell. The relation is the same as we saw before in the case of mitochondria. Just like mitochondria, chloroplasts were free-living microbes that stumbled upon the biotechnology of energy captured from a superior source.

In the case of mitochondria, I said that they found a way of burning their fuel in presence of oxygen which has many-fold higher energy yield than burning the food fuel in the absence of oxygen. In the case of chloroplast, they found a perennial source of energy in sunlight.

Making this even better is the fact that by doing photosynthesis, plants can degrade carbon dioxide, the product of oxygen metabolism, and regenerate oxygen. In other words, the plants re-synthesize oxygen from the waste product of higher energy-yielding oxygen technology.

Can you believe such monumentally important tasks are the handiwork of single-celled microbes?

One reason why I describe all this is to show that all microbes are not bad. The Corona virus experience twisted our view of the world of microbes. We may think, just like our immune system thinks, that all microbes are armed and dangerous.

It is high time to change this view.

To sum up, cyanobacteria (and later the chloroplast bacteria inside plant cells) gave us oxygen. The arrival of oxygen had the same impact on life systems as steel and coal had on the industrial revolution of our modern society.

The combustion engine that transformed the way we run our transportation was a direct beneficiary of this oxygen.

So, the microbial benevolence does not stop with the biotechnology of life systems, but also extended deep into the industrial technology.

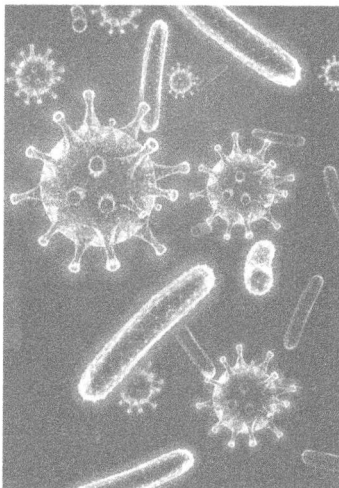

Chapter 17

THE DEPARTMENT OF IMMUNITY—OUR NATURAL WAY OF FIGHTING MICROBES

OUR DEPARTMENT OF IMMUNITY is broadly divided into two types. The first type is called Innate Immunity. The second type is called Adaptive Immunity.

The phrase *Innate Immunity* refers to intrinsic, non-specific, broad approaches to combating a microbial offender. It is like a street fight; combat between two people exchanging blows in unarmed brawls with clenched fists, wrenching teeth, boiling tempers, rapid heartbeats, breathlessness and flushed skin.

If you look at the animal kingdom, many animal species will exhibit more or less the same features while engaged in a tussle with their enemies. This is because these combat methods are chosen and selected by evolutionary forces and are retained across many animal species because they are fit for the purpose. There is no need to improve or lose them because they are good for defense. That is what innate defense tactics are all about.

129

When you take a look at our body's internal department of immunity certain defense and offense strategies are evolutionarily inherited by us as well as other life forms. This is like inherited wealth that your great grandfathers have left for you. Plants, fungi, insects, and other multi-cellular life forms all have great similarities in their innate immunity. Humans alone cannot claim ownership of the innate immunity tactics.

The adaptive immune system is different from the innate immune system. It is like the difference between a well-planned, orchestrated, organized attack on your enemies after studying them carefully versus a spur-of the moment fist fight on the street. In the latter what matters are raw emotions and use of conventional muscle power and you do not need to be trained for it. It comes as a natural gut instinct. In the former it is about planning and execution.

One of the common features of the innate immune defense across many life forms is the Complement System. It is a series of proteins all lined up in a functional cascade. For it to be fully functional the very first member of the complement cascade must be activated first. This activation is triggered by the offending microbe for example. Once the first member (C1) of the complement cascade is activated it activates the second protein member of the complement cascade. This goes on till the last member of the complement system (C9) is activated. One advantage of this type of cascade arrangement is that the effect of activation can be exponentially accelerated. As you go down the cascade there is an amplification of the activation in a quick timeframe.

Once fully activated the complement proteins C5-C9 combine and form a tubular structure that is hollow inside. What do we do with this tubular, molecular weapon that we assembled? We use it to stab the microbe to death. Yes, I am not joking. We stab the microbial guy till he bleeds dry and dies. The hollow nature of this molecular knife enables the internal contents of the microbe to flow out killing the microbe. What a cruel way to kill? Looking at it isn't it the way our human criminals kill their enemies?

Stabbing looks like a pretty crude way of killing someone. You are effectively making sure that you cut an artery or two so that the poor guy will lose all his blood until there is none left to transport oxygen and nutrients. It is a rather crude way of attacking an enemy when you are really intending to blockade the distribution systems of the body. Even slitting the throat is a horrifyingly crude way of killing by preventing intake of oxygen.

Somehow, the method of execution and the outcome don't seem to match in terms of sophistication. What I mean is that the intention of blockade of logistic operations inside the body sounds fancy, but the method used for that seems crude and unsophisticated. A knife-wielding criminal trying to kill someone seems like the last person in the world who knows that his intention was to cut off the energy supplies in the victim with a view to kill! To me he looks no more advanced than that Neolithic hunter that used a stone tool to clobber his victim. Maybe I can say that he rather looks like that Iron-age man who can use Iron for making his tool.

What do you do when you shoot a guy? You want him to bleed to death. For that you try to shoot at the heart so that all blood will gush out like we break a dam. The outcome you expect is the same as in the case of stabbing. Exsanguination is all about interfering with the global logistics of the body cells so that essential supplies are cut. The other outcome that you may expect is to puncture the lungs so that the guy will leak all the oxygen that he tries to bring in through the act of breathing. This has the same effect as attacking your gas or oil tankers.

You may try to look smarter than the yesteryear warriors or even criminals thinking that you are using technologically advanced weapons like guns and rifles rather than stones and knives. But the outcomes you hope to bring about are all about the interference in logistic supplies to the body cells. For that you are cutting open the arteries and puncturing the lungs like puncturing a car tire or something. Even within the immune system our innate defense tactic of the complement-mediated attack is designed like knifing where the complement complex punctures the cell wall of the microbe. What a tragedy? Can't we think of something more sophisticated than that? Are we still the cavemen who were using the barbaric, crude methods?

For that matter microbes adopt much more sophisticated ways of attacking us. As I said before, the Corona virus hacks your breathing apparatus without having to crudely puncture it like you do with your knife and guns. They use a much more delicate, refined method of inactivating your lungs so you can't breathe. To me the Corona virus looks far more sophisticated than humans in terms of attack capability.

The microbes also seem to know about this brutal knifing strategy. Amylocolaptosis is a type of bacteria which makes an antibiotic called Vancomycin for its own self-defense to protect itself against competing microbes. As usual we have exploited this Vancomycin antibiotic for our medical practice. In fact, Vancomycin is one of the antibiotics that are kept as a last straw in the fight against antibiotic resistance. This antibiotic is reserved for use against proven antibiotic-resistant bacteria. What is so special about Vancomycin? Vancomycin antibiotic molecule is a protein in nature and has a tubular, hollow structure very similar to the complement protein complex that we use to stab the microbes. The same way Amylocolaptosis bacteria use the Vancomycin protein knife to stab its enemy microbes.

This is what I said a little while ago. Similar primitive, innate methods of defense are widely prevalent across life forms.

Microbes are clever. When your department of immunity delivers a blow using the complement protein system they hit back. For example, a pathogenic bacterium like Pseudomonas attacks the first member of the complement cascade (C1) and destroys it. This prevents the activation of the complement system itself making it impossible for our immune system to use this tactic. Various other bacteria and some protozoa hit the complement system at various levels in the cascade with the same end result of inactivating this method of offense.

Microbes also use molecular mimicry i.e., similarity between their own molecules and that of the host, to evade the immune responses. Lipopolysaccharide (LPS), a type of endotoxin produced by Gram positive bacteria like Salmonella, Shigella, E. Coli and Neisseria meningitides, forms a confluent layer on the bacterial surface preventing complement-mediated cell lysis. I said earlier that complement activation is an important component of innate immunity. By coating themselves with the LPS coat the bacteria make themselves impenetrable by the complement-mediated attack. This is like wearing a bullet-proof jacket.

Neisseria gonorrhea, the bacteria that causes the sexually transmitted disease called Gonorrhea, can block complement activation by using the same LPS coat with a slight modification.

I mentioned streptococcus bacteria a little while ago. Its M protein binds the complement cascade control protein H of the host preventing its activation. This helps it escape the innate immune attack.

Some bacteria like S. pneumoniae, Candida albicans, E. histolytica produce a protein-destroying enzyme to degrade the complement C3 to escape the fury of the complement attack! As said before there are other microbes which dodge the complement system in various ways.

Moving on with other tactics used by our innate immunity let me describe the Natural Killer cell referred to as NK cells. This is not an imaginary name I have used to make it look interesting. This is the official name of a type of blood cell that works for the department of immunity. Its job is to kill the microbes like a trained assassin. In fact, these assassins specialize in virus attacks. How do they carry out their offensive against the viruses? They apparently target the body cells that are infected by the viruses. The NK cells destroy the body cells that are infected by the virus so that these viruses will be unable to keep spreading from one body cell to another. It is a questionable tactic because your virus-infected cells are destroyed. This may be viewed as anti-self and if something similar happened in our society human rights activists will have a field day trying to protest this. Fortunately, nature's laws are different, and this type of self-killing is allowed for the greater good.

There is another type of blood cell soldier who is enlisted

in the innate immunity battalion. He is called the Macrophage. The way the macrophage works is different. Macrophages engulf the microbial enemy and kill them by burning them in hell! Once engulfed, the microbial enemy is incarcerated for a period in one of the intracellular sacs called the lysosomes. Lysosomes are like the dungeons where prisoners are tortured to death. The microbe that was swallowed will be subjected to intense acidity and enzymatic degradation till death ensues.

It is worth noting that microbes can evade even this horrifying tactic. For example, the TB bacteria can hack the lysosome App and make it incapable of killing. Once it is done the TB bacteria can reside inside the macrophages for years without any questions asked. Then it slowly works its way towards destruction of the lungs. It is noteworthy that the microbes seem to prefer the lungs to kill. If you look at a lion or a tiger hunting down an animal, they will always go for the throat. The whole idea is to suffocate the animal to death. Microbes do the same. They target our breathing apparatus. Smartness of TB bacteria can be gathered in how effective they are in killing at least 5,000 people every single day for centuries running.

Neutrophils are another soldier class in the innate immunity division. They are white blood cells roaming the blood sea like our coast guards do. Neutrophils guard the blood sea 24/7. They don't sleep. In our daily lives it is common to injure ourselves with a minor cut here and there. At such times the microbes try to sneak into the blood surreptitiously. This is made easy by the gap in the skin fortress caused by the wound. Neutrophils rush to these troubled spots in no time. They stand guard against the microbial intruder. More neutrophil soldiers are recruited to the spot by signals sent out by the immune system. The neutrophils act like macrophages by swallowing the enemy and torturing them inside the cell by chemical methods.

Command codes are sent out by the immune system in the form of molecular signals to draw the neutrophils and macrophages to the scene of trouble. These codes guide the cells like a GPS system to the battle site. As you would expect, the enemy microbes seem to decode the signal codes sent out by our immune system and corrupt the signals. Or they destroy the code messages. This will prevent the cellular soldiers from being deployed. What a smart battle strategy? During the World War II it is said that three Polish mathematicians were used at Bletchley Park (UK) by the Allied Forces to decode the German Enigma codes. German Enigma machine used a very smart way of encoding their messages in billions of ways and they were proud that the enemies will never be able to break their codes. It was indeed cracked and that made German plans exposed and defeated. That is what the microbes do as well. They eavesdrop on what our immune soldiers communicate about the battle plans. They are as smart as us in communications and logistics.

I will mention one example. Our immune system makes antibodies (IgG) against the microbes which are used to attack them. One way the IgG antibody works is by facilitating the macrophage engulfment of the microbe. What do microbes do? Proteins A & G of Streptococci and S. aureus both bind and intercept the IgG directly preventing IgG-mediated phagocytosis. This is because of the molecular affinity between the bacterial proteins and our IgG antibodies. This means that the innate immunity department soldiers (like Macrophages) will become incapable of swallowing the microbial culprits.

Streptococcal bacteria have another trick up their sleeves. They make for themselves a sugar coat that resembles our own cell surface sugar coating. Because of this our immune cells are deceived into thinking that the streptococcal bacteria are probably our own.

The normal life span of these white blood cell soldiers is only 2-3 weeks. During times of immune wars their life span is even less. They die in action. The pus that you see in infected wounds is dead white blood cell soldiers who lost their lives in the service of your department of immunity. New white blood cells are produced in our bone marrow. Daily it is said that about 100 billion white blood cell soldiers are created. During times of infections this number will become 10 times more, it is said. That makes it 1 trillion cells a day. Imagine the cost of making so many new cells and what a drain this immune war is.

Another member of the innate immune system is the dendritic cell. These cells are located wherever our body is exposed freely to the outside environment. The idea is to guard these exposed areas. Typically, the exposed parts of our body include skin, windpipe, mouth and gut and even genitals. When a microbe tries to sneak in, these dendritic cells swallow them no different from the neutrophils and macrophages. One major difference is that dendritic cells swallow these microbes and disassemble them to decipher their features. Once they figure out their structure this is immediately conveyed to the Lymphocyte cell soldiers. In the language of immunity, a characteristic feature of a microbe that is a suitable target for the immune cells to attack is called an antigen. The immune system will generate custom-made defense weapons called antibodies that will be aimed like a directed missile at this antigen. It is the job of the dendritic cells to announce to the lymphocyte what the target antigens are on the enemy microbe. The lymphocyte cells upload this information in their database and they never forget it. Even if the microbe makes a re-entry after years the memory lymphocytes will recognize them and swing into action. In principle, this is no different from the criminal records held by our police forces on the criminals.

As previously stated, innate immune responses are seen in many different lifeforms. This includes the plants as well. Plants do not have a brain. They cannot move. They cannot social-distance themselves to escape from the microbes. They probably do not have something equivalent to our immune system. Certainly, they do not have an adaptive immune system like us. Adaptive immune system, as I said earlier, requires coordinated action of several defense cells. The plants don't have the concept of immune soldiers. But they do have defense mechanisms to protect against microbes. That is achieved by all plant cells having some sort of defense capabilities.

In the human immune system, some cells have microbe-detection systems. In general, recognition of microbes is achieved by sensing the antigens on their surface and this is done by receptors on our human T lymphocyte cell surfaces. It is called the T-cell antigen receptor (TCR). In the case of plants all plant cells have got the ability to pick up molecular signals from microbes once they have entered the plants. This is like having a local neighborhood watch where residents are empowered to keep an idea on intruders and once found they have a mechanism to communicate this information to rest of the residents. Our human immune system differs in that what we have is like having a full-fledged police force or even an army manned by trained, specialized people. Plant cells use their surface pattern recognition receptors to recognize microbe-associated molecular patterns and once found they immediately sound an alarm. They initiate a cascade of events that puts the plants in a defensive mode. They change from a growth mode to a defense mode.

I suppose the plant cell neighborhood watch is based on simple principles. If you found a man roaming around near your house wearing a hooded mask, it does not take a detective brain to conclude he is a thief. If you found a man running on the street with blood-stained clothes, then again you do not have to be Sherlock Homes to gather that a violent crime has been committed. Plants look for such simple tell-tale marks of the presence of an unwanted pathogen. This is based on something like behavioral pattern recognition that we do in our daily lives. The only difference is that the plants do the same using molecular pattern recognition (of the microbe).

Nature seems to allow co-evolution of lock and key alignment between the microbial surface molecules and the ones on the host cell surface enabling the microbes to enter and cause devastation. That sounds like cruelly one-sided favoritism, doesn't it?

Plants also look out for signs of damage to their body cells by sensing damage-associated molecular patterns to conclude the need for action. If you find a car or a house damaged in your neighborhood, then you suspect the presence of some miscreants and you take extra care or alert the police and fellow residents. If the damage extends to more properties, then your response will be much more. Plants can do the same. They can assess the damage to their cells through the signals emitted by damaged plant cells. Once found they activate a process by which the plants will start making molecules called disease resistance factors whose job is to combat the pathogen-secreted toxins. They do by activating programmed cell death at the infected plant sites so that the infection will not further spread. The plants also produce molecular signals like methyl salicylic acid and azelaic acid which are transported from infected sites to non-infected sites. Once these signals are received the yet-to-be-infected plant sites start their defense mechanisms which include production of agents with anti-microbial activity.

Plants have a unique mechanism to fight viruses. They target the RNA operating system of the viruses and silence them! This is called RNA silencing. This makes the viruses starve of genetic code information and die. Now it's the turn of the plants to act like Bletchley Park mathematicians to decode the viral enigma codes.

RNA silencing has emerged as a useful scientific method used by researchers to study genes. They have copied the plant technology (which is not unusual for humans) to inactivate RNAs decoded from certain genes whose function we do not know yet. By doing so the gene's function will be forcibly lost and the effects of it will give us an idea what was that lost function which was mediated by the gene.

Some RNA viruses have evolved evasive strategies to beat the RNA silencing defense. What they do is transform their RNA operating system to the DNA form using reverse transcriptase enzymes. HIV virus is a classic example. By converting their codes into the DNA form (the same form used by humans) they manage to integrate their codes into the human codes. Once integrated our immune cells can no longer distinguish between our own gene codes and that of the virus and there escapes the virus. When you are looking for a criminal the last place you will look for is the police station. The virus does exactly that. They hide in a place where you will never look for them.

Even microbes have these kinds of innate immune responses. I said before that there are viruses called

Bacteriophages which infect the bacteria and kill them. What do the bacteria do? They use a molecular saw to cut the RNA code string of the virus. The molecular saw the bacteria use is an enzyme. It is called the Restriction Endonuclease. This enzyme helps to physically cut the viral RNA codes like someone slitting the throat. What a gruesome yet digital strategy? Readers may wonder if I am using my imagination to concoct science fiction stories, but I am not. The microbes are hackers to the core.

I mentioned the dramatic impact this microbial technology of restriction endonuclease has had on one of the most important medical and scientific revolutions called Genetic Engineering! Genetic Engineering and all the huge advances man has had because of this technology would never have happened if only the microbes did not lend their technology (free of cost with no intellectual property payments).

I also mentioned earlier another bacterial cyber technology of gene cutting in the form of CRISPR enzymes. This technique has already been borrowed heavily by the human scientific fraternity just as they did with the restriction endonuclease.

Let us now move on to the other arm of the department of Immunity Adaptive Immunity. The Lymphocyte white blood cells are the soldiers of the Adaptive Immune system. There are two types of lymphocytes B and T. Both have different strategies to deal with microbial enemies. These strategies are based on one common thing a customized attack on the offenders. This is something unique about our immune system. We just do not use the same strategy fits all approach when fighting the bacteria and viruses.

Once a microbial intruder is identified by our immune system the B lymphocytes make a custom-tailored antibody targeted against the microbe. A surface component of the microbe will be selected as the target. This is like making a custom-made bullet for your gun each time you want to hit your enemy. These antibody bullets are made within 7-10 days after the entry of the microbe. As I said before the microbe tries to evade the antibody bullets by tucking in their surface component against which the antibody bullets are fired. In other instances, like in the case of Staphylococcus bacteria, the escape from the antibody can be accomplished by the microbe by coating themselves with some host components like fibrin. This conceals microbial target from the antibody.

There are bacteria and viruses that can change the nature and appearance of their surface during the infection. This is like wearing a disguise. When the antigenic molecules on the surface of the microbe change, the immune system needs more time to work on customizing to the newly changed target. Because the target keeps changing our antibodies become useless or less effective while the microbes march on undisturbed. In some cases, like the Cholera bacteria, Typhoid bacteria, Streptococcus bacteria (the one that causes skin infections and pneumonia) etc. there are many types of variants that have evolved and become fixed as permanent variations. There are over one hundred types of the Streptococcus bacteria that cause pneumonia. There are over 80 types of the same bacteria that cause skin infections. The emergence of so many types of the same microbial species means that they have multiplied their chances of beating our immune system. Just to fight the streptococcus bacteria, we can make at least 180 types of antibody responses and you can imagine the strain it will produce on our immune system.

Some microbial pathogens like Shigella, Listeria and E. coli can take up intracellular locations and essentially hide from the surveillance of the B and T lymphocyte soldiers. The antibody bullets can't hit something that is hiding inside our own cells.

Tests for diagnosis of infections include basically two types. The first type is detection of antibodies in the blood directed against the microbe. Because the antibodies are specific for each type of microbe there are individual tests available for each type of microbe. The presence of an antibody against a specific microbe is evidence that the person has been previously exposed to the microbe. This is like circumstantial evidence collected during investigation of a crime. When someone is showing signs of an infection, the doctor becomes a sleuth combing the patient's body for evidence that will throw light on the microbial criminal. The presence of antibody in the patient's blood is like finding the fingerprints on the scene of crime. One shortcoming of the antibody test is that we cannot pinpoint the time of occurrence of the microbial crime. This is because the antibodies stay in the blood stream for months and years after the microbe had committed the crime.

The second type of test used in diagnosis of a microbial infection is the PCR test (Polymerase Chain Reaction). This test looks for the presence of microbial RNA or DNA codes circulating in the patient's body. One advantage of this PCR test is that it can pick up the microbial offender almost in real-time even as the offense is being committed. The doctors can arrive at the crime scene while the crime is in progress. It is a different matter altogether that they are unable to do much about it if the criminals are viruses. This is because we have not got any effective treatment for them. Even bacterial criminals often give the slip and complete the crime because in many cases they can evade our antibiotic shootings.

Our adaptive immune system relies on several other molecular weapons in addition to the antibodies. They are all manufactured by lymphocyte soldiers. When you talk of arms manufacturing in the real world it is done by big corporations in facilities that take millions to build. Then there are these arms dealers as well. But, inside your body arms manufacturing is a DIY job! Can you believe that? Soldiers make their own weapons! This is inconceivable by any stretch of imagination in our so-called modern society.

The weapons made by the lymphocytes are Interleukins and Interferons. There are many types of them. Each of those sub-types has specific functions. It would be boring to go through each one of them and so I am going to refrain from doing so. It is okay if I am writing a textbook, but I am not writing a textbook here. Interferon Gamma is one such molecular weapon coming under the Interferon class of ammunition. These are very effective against viruses. You guessed it right. Viruses like the Flu virus and the Dengue fever virus thwart the Interferon Gamma attack by hitting the manufacturing operations inside the lymphocytes. That is ingenious, isn't it? It saves the trouble of fighting the lymphocytes and its weapons. This is a highly cost-effective battle strategy.

Lymphocyte soldiers are normally patrolling the blood sea like the Coast Guards I said. They are also stationed in regional bases much like what we do. US, for example, have numerous naval bases dotted around the world in strategic locations. This allows the rapid deployment of troops to locations where conflicts happen. If they relied on troops stationed in the US they would not be able to respond in time to aggressions from their enemies. The same way the lymphocytes are also stationed in regional bases called the Lymph Nodes. They are in every sense of the word like our military bases that we see in the real world. Lymphocytes troops can be dispatched to troubled locations in the body in no time. Lymph nodes are distributed all around our body. They are pea-sized glands. You can find them in your neck, axilla, and inguinal regions apart from some internal organ locations. These nodes swell up during times of strife. That indicates rapid multiplication of lymphocyte soldiers to meet the demands. When you have an infection in your body the nearest lymph nodes will swell up and become palpable. Doctors look for inflamed nodes to detect signs of microbial intrusion. If you had an infection in your mouth, then the nodes in your neck region will become inflamed. Even tonsil glands are like the lymph nodes because immune cells are stationed here too. Tonsils are located tight at the entry point of the food pipe and by virtue of its strategic location it is guarding a vital point. Inflammation of the tonsils is a common phenomenon for which we seek medical attention. What do doctors do? They usually remove the inflamed tonsil which, when you think of it, is antagonistic to the natural defense mechanism of your body. This is like using the anti-inflammatory drugs to curtail the natural immune reactions our body initiates. It occurs as though medical practitioners are anti-nature.

One impressive feature of our adaptive immune system is that it can devise an attack strategy to any unknown microbe even if that microbe is totally new to the planet Earth. Immunology textbooks clearly mention that the B lymphocytes will rearrange their antibody gene codes to customize an attack against a microbial offender even if it is totally new to mankind. I am not writing a sci-fi book, but I am not the first one to say that we can initiate an immunological defense against any microbe in the universe! Readers who had studied Biochemistry or Immunology may well remember the chapter in Immunology textbooks on antibody genes and their structure. B lymphocytes create new antibody genes by permutation and combination of the antibody gene components. An average individual can make at least 100 billion types of antibodies! Can you imagine one single cell class (B lymphocytes) having the ability to create that level of diversity?

Our human cells have about 30,000 genes only. Antibody production is one of the multitudes of functions carried out by the genes. We expect some genes to be devoted to this important role. If we relied on preset, ready-made antibody genes then there would be a limitation on the number antibodies you can make. Even if you considered an unlikely scenario of allocating all genes for antibody production then the maximum number of antibodies you can make is going to be less than 30,000 only.

Then why do we have an antibody repertoire said to exceed 100 billion? This is because evolution designed a better system. It keeps a finite number of antibody components to be mixed and matched as required. This way it's possible to create an infinite variety. This design enables us to be prepared for new microbes that keep evolving. As I said earlier, viruses evolve rapidly, and we cannot be left defenseless. We need systematic capability to assemble a solution as rapidly as possible.

This system is like cooking. We use a finite number of cooking ingredients, but the number of worldwide culinary recipes far exceeds that number. This is achieved by various combinations of the cooking ingredients and preparation methods.

A better example is the art of writing and how humanity generated an infinite number of books using just 26 letters. We rearrange letters in grammatically allowed ways and there appear endless number of books, magazines and essays.

Digital technology goes further. Binary codes are just two (0 and 1). But look at the number of gadgets out there.

The ability to make over 100 billion types of antibody bullets sounds impressive. The number of types of microbes on the planet may be much less than that number. There are about 300,000 types of viruses out there though we know only about 6500 of them. It is even better that only about 200 of them really infect humans. In terms of bacteria, it is said there are about 30,000 types of bacteria out there. The number of bacterial types that can infect humans will be far less. Given the relatively miniscule numbers of microbes that can attack us it is clear that our antibody bullet repertoire is excessively well-equipped. May be that is why they say that we are prepared for microbes coming from even a faraway world.

What I want to add here is that whatever we try to come up with the microbe is not going to just fall dead. They will fight back. Fighting back is a birthright for all life forms on the planet. Even the most sophisticated immune weapon your body makes will find stiff resistance from your microbial enemies. They will find a way out. Time and again this is proven beyond doubt.

Interestingly, all the things that I discussed so far about our immune system and the way the microbes evade these immune attacks are all happening at a cellular level without any input whatsoever from the thinking faculty of a brain. This is the most surprising part. This includes even the offensive strategies used by the microbes. Nowhere do we find highly paid executives, bureaucrats, scientists and advisors doing the brainstorming. Yet, we find unbelievable things happen.

If man stopped fighting with his own species and focused more on fighting the real enemies such as microbes, then I am sure he would do far better than he is doing now. Enormous resources are spent on fighting wars with nations and very little for fighting the immune wars. No other species on the planet is as senseless as us. Especially the organisms without brains are the ones who seem to be doing fine in terms of internal peace. The brain probably messes things up by allowing irrelevant factors like ego and greed to come into the picture.

Not all microbes are our enemies though. There are some who do good for us. We cannot live without them. They are that good.

Microbes are, in my opinion, biological applications written using gene codes. They have their roles to play in our lives. The types of biological actions carried out by microbes clearly suggest that they are created for a purpose. I am convinced of that. I do not think microbes exist just for the purpose of infecting us and causing misery. I suppose one reasoning behind this phenomenon could be cybernetic control on density of our population. I will not rule out the possibility that microbes are here to keep our population under check. We may have temporarily overcome this microbial feedback loop on human mortality rates by our medical advances, but I repeatedly mentioned how the microbes are conquering us by resistance to antibiotics. Viruses have always been carrying out their business unhindered by medical sciences. Of course, the vaccines like smallpox vaccine, Polio vaccine, Measles vaccine etc. have played a big role in creating herd immunity and protecting us. But we have a long way to go. Viruses like the AIDS virus and the Corona virus are rude wake up calls that remind us we are not as powerful as we think.

As a life system, they have the same right as you to live on Earth. They could employ any means at their disposal to accomplish the objective of survival. They need to survive to fulfill their biological roles.

Everything on the planet exists for a reason.

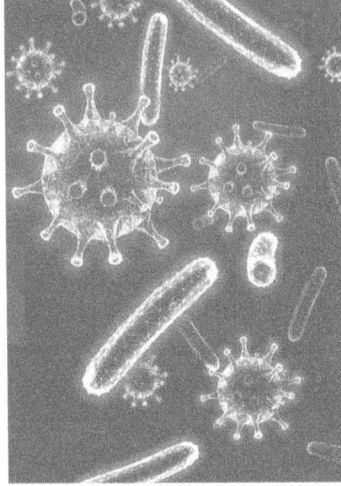

Chapter 18

ORIGIN OF VIRUSES, SELFISH GENES AND THE GENETIC ARMS RACE

VIRUSES ARE THE most populous of all creatures on Planet Earth and do not even figure in the classification scheme of life.

Life forms are classified (called Taxonomy) according to a simple system devised by the Swedish Botanist Carolus Linnaeus in the 18th century. Microbes fall under the domains of Archaea, Eubacteria and few under Eukaryote. The next level of hierarchy is the Kingdom where microbes nicely fit in the groups Fungi, Protista and Archaebacteria. Thus, bacteria, fungi, algae and protozoa are present in the Tree of Life. But viruses are not accounted for. They are simply not mentioned or included in the three life domains.

This is surprising.

Perhaps the reason viruses are not included in the Life category is they are not alive. Or viruses could be viewed as something that is between Life and Non-life.

Why are viruses considered non-living? This may be because viruses cannot live on their own without a host organism supporting them. They cannot generate metabolic energy because they don't have the necessary cellular structures. They cannot make copies of themselves unless they borrow Ribosomes, the protein-synthesizing factory of the host cells. In other words, they cannot reproduce without the host's help. If something cannot reproduce on their own, they cannot be given the status of living beings.

The origin of life probably started with one important step. That step was the formation of an enclosing membrane that apportioned a little atomic matter inside each vesicle. This vital piece of biological construction is akin to a house construction. Your house separates your family from the street. It is the enclosing membrane that separates cellular contents from the environment.

If this membrane did not form, then everything would be part of the whole environment and we would not have localized life forms. An average prokaryotic life form (single-celled) is only about 0.1 to 5 microns in diameter. That is small—a meter divided in a million portions is 1 micron!

What could be held inside such a small sac measuring a millionth of a meter? The prokaryotic bacteria don't appear to be greedy at all. They are satisfied with the amount of matter that can be packed inside a vesicle this small. We human beings are packed in a body bag measuring on average 1.6 meters tall which is about 1.6 million times longer than a bacterium.

One may wonder why would, or rather how would, a membrane form encircling a piece of lifeless, atomic matter? I have always had this doubt. This is the single most important step in the formation of life. For this step, what was needed was a bit of fatty stuff. Look at a cup of milk. What was liquid soon forms a layer of membrane on its surface. This happens with an oil-rich gravy, too, because the fat content inside the milk or the oily gravy floats to the top and the fatty molecules align with each other due to their chemical affinity.

Something similar happened almost 3.5 billion years ago in

the primordial earth. For that to happen some amount of atomic evolution must have preceded that allowed formation of different sorts of molecules like RNA/DNA, amino acids and particularly fats.

Strangely, some viruses like Adenovirus and Papillioma virus do not have a cell envelope. They belong to the class of non-enveloped viruses. The fact that they do not have an enclosing membrane adds weight to the argument that viruses are not living creatures. They could be considered in the same class of lifeless entities like grains of sand.

In 2013, virologists Chantal Abergel and Jean-Michel Claverie from the Aix-Marseille University, discovered the largest virus of them all in a sample of dirt collected from Siberia. This virus had remained there for over 30,000 years. This virus was named Pithovirus. It was more massive than even some bacteria.

While small viruses have as few as 4 genes, this Pithovirus had well over 500 genes. Some of these genes were used for complex tasks such as making proteins and repairing and replicating DNA. These are functions not normally associated with viruses which are considered incapable of independently carrying out these functions without the help from a host cell. While most viruses hijacked host cell machinery for these functions the Pithovirus was different.

Generally, viruses are believed to have arisen after proto-life forms appeared with the basic structure of enclosed space (membrane-bound). In other words, viruses could not have preceded the origin of cellular life forms. As I said earlier, early Earth was basically composed of atoms. There were no complex molecules yet. It took some time for them to form.

The famous Stanley Miller and Harold Urey experiment performed in 1952 at the University of Chicago showed how the primitive Earth harbored basic, simple chemicals that could transform to complex molecules like amino acids, DNA bases, etc. Charles Darwin called the Earth a warm little pond where life formed and evolved.

It is said that the early Earth saw that big step of formation of enclosed spaces we call cells. Without this step there was no way individual lifeforms could originate. If the majority view that viruses need a host to parasitize, then that requires the world to have become cell-rich. Only then could viruses form. This assumption is based on virus dependency on host cells. So, viruses could not have formed on Earth before the formation of cellular life.

Origin of Life theorists propose a scenario wherein early proto-life cells subsequently evolved over an undisclosed period to form what is called the Last Universal Common Ancestor (LUCA) which subsequently diversified into the modern cells leading to the three super-kingdoms: Archaea, Bacteria and Eukarya. The question is whether the viruses came before or after the LUCA.

Genomes of archaeoviruses, bacterioviruses and eukaryoviruses (i.e., viruses that infect members of these domains Archaea, Bacteria and Eukaryote) are characterized by abundance of virus-specific genes that lack detectable similarities in cellular genomes (i.e., genes of host cells). The existence and abundance of diverse virus groups suggests they probably started very early in evolution. The viral lineages infecting distantly related hosts from all the three super-kingdoms share several conserved protein folding structures that also indicate that these viral lineages existed prior to the LUCA origin and diversification.

If we entertain the theory that ancient proto-cells evolved into viruses (before or after the origin of LUCA), then we should consider the possibility that viral nucleic acids first evolved in the pre-cellular world. Then viral propagation methods evolved via the modification of the cellular proteins to function as viral capsids once cells appeared via evolution. Viral capsids are like the cell membranes we talked about earlier. The only difference is that these viral capsids are made of proteins and not fats.

There is a big question about viruses and their putative origins. The question is: do they evolve bigger by robbing genes from hosts? Or do they simply evolve like any other organism by replication and mutations?

Viruses may have overdone the reduction part because they also shed the ability to make energy, or the ability to make proteins, and even the ability to make copies (reproduction). If viruses originated after the origin of cellular life (which can serve the function of a host) then it makes sense that viruses took a lean and mean approach to survival. But if the viruses originated before cellular life forms, then the story of viruses and their lifestyle does not add up. If there were no cellular hosts, then what could they parasitize?

Another point worth noting in the gigantic viruses like Pithovirus and Pandoravirus is that many of their genes do not have counterparts in standard life forms. This means their genes are unique and may have evolved independently.

This finding throws new light on the origins of viruses—they might have originated and descended from unique ancestors separate and different from the cellular life forms. Their origins may have been independent events not dependent on cellular life.

Apart from the types of genes and the similarities between viral and cellular counterparts, another striking difference found in some of these big viruses is their proteins fold differently in a 3-D shape. Protein-folding is how a strip of amino acids eventually exist in 3-D forms. Amino acids can fold in unpredictable ways. There are characteristic patterns of folding seen in standard lifeforms, but in these big viruses, the folding can be different—meaning they come from a separate lineage.

Many researchers take the view that viruses, particularly the ones with DNA as the operating system instead of RNA, evolved from one or multiple ancient cells (primordial lifeforms) via deliberate reduction (i.e., downsizing of genes and size). Considering the unique composition of the viral genomes, this model better fits the evolutionary biology of parasitic and endo-symbiotic organisms.

The survival benefits of parasitism and propagation via release of viral particles may have selected this type of lifeform which now haunts us in various sizes and forms including

COVID-19—which is by no means the first or the last of the viruses to cause nuisance to Home sapiens.

It is loosely said that viruses steal our genes and use them for their survival, but many virologists argue differently. Since the total number of viruses far outweighs the other life systems, even with a small number of genes, the total number of viral genes outnumbers host gene numbers in the biosphere. Novel viral genes continuously arise during replication and recombination of viral genomes.

A survival strategy of the viruses involves transfer and integration of viral genes into the host genome. Retroviruses (such as the AIDS virus) are classical examples of this type of gene transfer from the virus to the host (not the other way).

These viral genes become part of the host cell genes and incredibly, they might become functional. Even more incredible is the fact that these viral genes can benefit the host. 8% of the human genome is derived from over 100,000 retroviral gene fossils. The word fossil is used here in the sense that this integration of the retroviral viral genes happened long ago in the distant past and we humans still carry them around like baggage, functional or not.

If these viral genes were integrated in germ cells, then we even pass them down to generations vertically. Sequencing the genomes of multiple animal species shows that multiple non-retroviral gene fossils are still remnant.

Along with his colleagues, Maulik Patel from Fred Hutchinson Cancer Research Center in the US wrote a review article in the journal Current Opinion in Virology in 2011 titled *Paleovirology—ghosts and gifts of viruses past*. They argue that many viral genes end up serving the host life system for housekeeping or defense functions. In some cases, they may be used to interfere with virus-virus communications or virus-host exchanges.

Viruses that lived millions of years ago seem to have invaded the genomes of early life forms that existed at that time. The retroviruses had the ability to enter the personal space of the host organisms by stitching their DNA to that of the host.

This may not have been easily tolerated by the early host organisms and they might have developed ways of defending their integrity. Over time the integrated viral genes probably did their bit of harm as they still do. The hosts might still be learning to cope with this menace. Patel and his colleagues refer to this as the evolutionary echoes of ancient conflicts. The surprising thing here is that these viral genes may have become inactive or recycled by the host towards some useful host functions. Or, even worse, these viral genes could cause disease.

An example of a viral gene being used by placental mammals is the syncitin gene which was inserted into primate genomes allegedly 35 million years ago. Primates evolved to use this viral gene for trophoblast development in the placenta meaning a virus contributed to the evolution of the reproductive function in placental mammals.

Friend-virus susceptibility -1 or Fv1 gene is another example of a retroviral gene domesticated by higher organisms. This gene is derived from the retroviral Gag gene and is estimated to have been inserted into host cells 7 million years ago. This viral-origin gene plays a role as an antiviral factor suggesting hosts could use viral genes for interfering with virus-virus or virus-host interactions so successful viral infection does not take place.

Paleo virology is a field where scientists study viral remnants, active or inactive, in host genomes. Just as archeologists use dating methods to estimate the age of unearthed items, these paleo virologists try to pinpoint the time viruses transferred their genes to the hosts.

These genes may persist in the same form or in a mutated form. They may have become dormant or inactive. They may have also become a part of the host genomes contributing functionally. New methods for database searches are needed to identify virus-related gene sequences in higher organisms.

Current methods for analyzing such genes may not bear fruit if the gene sequence is entirely new and might not have a counterpart in other organisms. As of now, many animal genomes have large amounts of gene sequences that don't belong. Perhaps these alien gene sequences were inserted by a virus in ancient times.

Some people assume technologies came from alien civilizations if they are considered far ahead of the times. For example, the Egyptian pyramids were built with such amazing precision following advanced geometric principles. Everyone knows human civilization did not have the necessary technology to build such structures 5,000 years ago. Then who built them?

There was never stone-based technology before this period, and it is difficult to believe the very first stone architecture built by man is so gigantic and cannot be reproduced until this day. So, we implicate aliens. In the same way, many of the gene sequences in higher animals are not fully understood in terms of their origins and function. Paleo virologists implicate ancient viruses, and it is difficult to refute their argument.

Patel and his colleagues use the word *domestication* of the viral genes by the host life system which is a very novel idea. It is like what countries do in military intelligence. Countries get the blueprints of novel military gadgets from the enemies through espionage and use the design for making more or even to improve upon them.

Business enterprises are known to use elements of designs from competitors for the betterment of their products. In other words, viruses seem to be able to influence host biology. Several documented cases exist which clearly show that viruses were involved in the emergence of evolutionary innovations. The idea that gene flux from viruses to a host's life systems is overwhelmingly more than expected. This suggests we should view viruses in a totally different light.

The New York Times carried a news article on 4 October 2017 written by Carl Zimmer titled *Ancient Viruses are buried in your DNA*. Basically, this is the paleo virology I referred to. Some of these ancient viruses—or their relics—may protect us from disease or make us prone to diseases like cancer. The interesting thing is that most of these buried viral genes are from retroviruses which invaded our genomes, or that of other lifeforms. millions of years ago. They are grouped together and referred to as Endogenous Retroviruses (ERVs).

Dr. Odile Heidmann, a French researcher, published a finding in 2017 wherein a protein encoded by a viral gene embedded in our genome (due to a Retroviral invasion that happened about 100 million years ago) is secreted by the fetus into the maternal blood stream. This viral gene is conserved across many species—which suggests it is not a relic but has important functions. It is supposed to code for a retroviral envelope. She hypothesized that this virally encoded Hemo protein could be a message from the fetus to the mother dampening the mother's immune system, so it does not attack the fetus. What could be the relation between a gene that codes for a retroviral envelope and mammalian reproduction? This Hemo protein gene is expressed from placenta suggesting a role in reproduction.

This Hemo protein is also expressed in the placenta, stem cells and even in some tumors. This team of researchers suggested this protein could also determine if a cell can assume an all-rounder capability which means it takes the cell back in time when the cell was a Stem cell.

A Stem cell is one which is still not differentiated.

During embryonic growth, all our cells are like this—they are undifferentiated into individual cell types. They are like school children that have the potential to become what they want to be. The children could study to become doctors, engineers, lawyers, businessman or athletes. They study the proper courses to reach their chosen profession. They know this is a long process and an irreversible one at that. Few doctors decide to change professions and become a lawyer or engineer. Few lawyers decide to become engineers. It's possible, impractical. I would be surprised if one in a million lawyers ever did that.

Professional specialization is like cellular differentiation in biology. Cells are alike in the embryonic stage. They are all like school children bubbling with the potential to become specialized in a chosen path: a kidney cell, a brain cell, a muscle cell or a blood cell, etc. No kidney cell retraces its path to a stem cell. No kidney cell becomes a muscle cell or vice versa. Cellular differentiation is like school children getting educated.

What I am trying to say is that this irreversible path of cellular specialization can be reversed under some circumstances. This typically happens in cancerous conditions. A cancer cell typically loses its specialized status and assumes the primitive, undifferentiated state. The more undifferentiated they become the more aggressive they grow. Losing their differentiation and specialization makes them capable of dividing and multiplying more. That is the advantage the cancer cells gain by losing their specialized status.

Odile Heidmann and colleagues in their paper on Hemo protein suggested that expression of this protein somehow helps to take the cells back in time to the stage of undifferentiated stem cell status. By doing so, the cells may assume a cancerous state. That is why may be this Hemo protein was found to be expressed in many types of cancers in humans.

The other point is that Hemo protein may also drive the cells towards undifferentiated stem cell status that prevails in embryonic growth. I mentioned another retroviral gene relic called the Syncitin gene that assumes a host role in development of trophoblast maturation and placental growth. Hemo protein shares some of the properties of Syncitins but is different because it is secreted and shed in the extracellular environment (in this case mother's blood stream). Because the Hemo protein is expressed from the 8-cell stage in the embryo and persists until all stages of embryonic growth it can be safely said that it has a role to play in the development of the fetus.

Hemo protein gene could also play a role in other functions. A protective role against infection by other viruses/retroviruses is also hypothesized. Because the product of this gene is the retroviral envelope, it is possible the secreted envelope protein could act as a decoy for real viruses to bind to, thereby preventing attachment of the virus to host tissues for colonization.

Robin Weiss wrote an article titled *Human endogenous retroviruses: friend or foe* in a microbiology journal in January 2016 where he summarized the current knowledge about these embedded viral genes. In this article, he says Charles Darwin may be intrigued to know that viruses may have been influential in our evolution—not just monkeys.

It is likely these retroviruses etched a symbiotic relationship with us and other animals by integrating themselves into the host DNA. As can be expected of any symbiotic relationship, both parties have a reciprocal give and take arrangement. We do not fully understand the mechanisms behind these interactions.

Endogenous retroviruses are present in all phyla of vertebrates ranging from cartilaginous fish to mammals and birds. Beyond retroviruses, herpes virus genomes are also seen in 0.8% of Caucasian population integrated at the tail ends of the chromosomes.

Virus-Host interaction is a theme permeating the entire course of life's evolution. This interaction is commonly pictured as an arms race where hosts constantly evolve new means of defense while viruses perpetually evolve to evade, as written by Eugene Koonin and Valerian Dolja in their review article titled *A virocentric perspective on the evolution of life* published in October 2013.

It is not just viruses that hijack host genes for counter-defense and other functions. Hosts also routinely recruit viral genes for diverse roles about which we are only starting to learn. Given their high rates of mutation and evolution, viruses might comprise the principal source of novel genes in the biosphere. If that is the case, what is the problem in borrowing some genes from them?

Koonin and Dolija call viruses nature's genomic laboratory. Most organisms use either DNA or RNA as their operating systems. Viruses exploit all forms of nucleic acids single-stranded or double-stranded, RNA or DNA, RNA that can be converted to DNA as in retroviruses, linear or circular RNA and DNA, protein-linked RNA or DNA, etc.

In addition, they have diverse replication-expression strategies. The genetic diversity of viruses is no less startling than their physical abundance. It is said that much of the viral gene sequences are dark matter, about which we do not understand. This is because there are no equivalents of these gene sequences in other life forms. The seemingly unlimited diversity of viral genes contrasts with other life systems who generally have a substantial number of common genes between them.

It is likely that viruses represent the principal reservoir of genetic diversity on earth. Most viral genes are not widespread and are poorly conserved. Yet, there are some viral hallmark genes shared by a wide range of viruses that code for the essential vital functions—including the capsid proteins, RNA or DNA replicating enzymes, integrase enzymes that help in insertion of viral genes into the host, etc. The smallest virus genomes consist mostly of these hallmark genes while in the large viruses these hallmark genes are only a minority. Some bacteriophages and archaeal viruses lack hallmark genes— replaced by identifiable substitutions with functionally similar host-derived genes.

It is alleged that evolution of life started with a virus-like stage with the appearance of cellular life forms much later. These early life forms (or proto-life forms) that were the precursors of viruses used capsid protein envelopes to delineate each virion.

As well, there were viral forms that lacked capsid envelope and we see them even today. The icosahedral viral capsid protein model is seen in diverse viruses infecting bacteria, Archaea and eukaryotes. It is true that numerous different types of capsid proteins exist and make up this unusual geometric structure that more looks like an alien space craft. The later cellular life forms used a fatty envelope apart from relying on ribosomes for translation of the genomic information. The latter feature was lacking in the early viruses, and this continues today.

The virus world can be seen as being composed of selfish genetic elements, capsid-covered or not. These selfish gene elements go to any length to propagate themselves. This is in line with the Selfish Gene hypothesis put forward by Richard Dawkins. He argued in his much-acclaimed book that the purpose of life is to ensure the genes survive. This contradicts the traditional view that the purpose of life is to survive and reproduce at the organismal level. The molecules that formed in the primordial soup that existed in the earth's early environment soon progressed towards a replicator copies these molecules, i.e., the genes.

All organisms employ multilayered systems of defense against invasion of foreign genetic material. This invasion comes from viruses or other selfish gene elements. Cellular organisms evolved strategies to detect this invasion and eliminate the newly added gene sequences from the original content. Failure to do so results in contamination of gene sequences coming from foreign gene invaders. Genes must protect themselves against this onslaught.

In primordial times, genes evolved out of the inorganic environment that prevailed then. A lot of pre-cellular evolution happened over many million years where this primordial pool of genes mixed and inter-mixed with others that had also spontaneously formed under the influence of the organizing principles that existed on the primordial earth.

As many readers know, Stanley and Miller's experiment proved that if you provide a mix of basic chemical elements and a source of energy and water, then complex biomolecules like amino acids and building blocks of DNA/RNA like purine and pyrimidine form as if by magic.

This is proven science.

In fact, this is also proven by analysis of meteorites such as the Mutchison meteorite that fell on Australia in 1969. It was supposed to have formed almost 7 billion years ago. That means this meteorite formed 2.5 billion years before the earth formed. It must have circulated the solar system for all this time.

Scientists analyzed the composition of this meteorite to see if it contained organic molecules. This offered convincing proof that life-sustaining biomolecules can form spontaneously anywhere else in the Solar system—just as they formed on our nascent earth.

As expected, more than 14,000 types of biomolecules were found embedded in the meteorite. It had many types of amino acids, hydrocarbons (fats), nucleic acid bases and a whole lot of others. They must have formed deep in interstellar space from inorganic elements lurking in gaseous clouds. This is the same process that happened on earth.

The nature of atoms and molecules makes them sticky by default. Their chemical and physical affinity for binding and bonding with other chemical moieties makes them stick to each other—which naturally builds more complex molecular structures. Infinite numbers of permutations and combinations allow the buildup of complexity without having to invoke any divine influences.

As atoms and molecules form higher order structures, emergent properties manifest. What does this mean? This means that newer properties are conferred on molecular assemblies that are more than the sum of the individual properties of each molecule constituent.

A simple example is salt. Sodium and chloride atoms together form salt. The salty taste that you get is not inherently present in either sodium or chlorine.

More important things can happen too. Amino acids, which form spontaneously in inorganic environments, are like the alphabets of proteins. Assembling amino acids to get different kinds of proteins is like writing sentences using an alphabet. Left alone over time, individual amino acids naturally bind and bond with other compatible amino acids following the grammar of chemistry.

You would not write sentences using random words. Because grammar demands it, some words are preceded or followed by other words. In the same way, alphabets create words. For example, I do not know a word where the letter Z follows the letter L—or vice versa. Whereas some letters like A will be followed by lots of other letters. I hope you see what I mean.

In the same way, the chemical moieties of atoms and molecules have preferred affinities and repulsions. This is based purely on their chemistry. This is like people forming relationships with others affinity,

Creating proteins from naturally formed amino acids was a

phenomenally important step in the origin of life. Without proteins, there is no life because proteins are the molecular engineers who support life. One of the striking emergent properties caused by a protein is catalysis. Catalysis means execution of a molecular or cellular task in a simpler and facilitated manner. For example, enzymes are proteins with the emergent property of catalysis. Proteins can also assume structural or other functional roles. For example, one of the earliest life-sustaining proteins that evolved was the ATP-synthesizing enzyme in cellular power plants: mitochondria. This made energy capture possible—the energy required for cell function.

Over millions of years, inorganic elements spewed from faraway stars and gathered in nebulous gas clouds. They clumped together as earth in a process no different from any other planet's formation. As chemical interactions built up, more complex molecules began to form. Interesting things happened when raw materials formed nucleic acids. Nucleic acids are RNA or DNA. They use purine and pyrimidine bases as building blocks and are the equivalent of amino acids, the building blocks of proteins.

Purine and pyrimidine bases are the alphabets used to write gene sentences. From random interactions, purine or pyrimidine bases formed linear strands. When a lot of these DNA/RNA alphabets were assembled in a stretch they acquired meaning. They were like a collection of pre-defined sequences of alphabets conveying meaning. The only difference is that nobody sat and wrote these DNA or RNA sequences—they formed from random processes.

As a result, one thing that happened from the assembly of the nucleic acid bases was emergence of the property of execution. The word execution refers to the property of directed control. In IT parlance this is called Executable code. What was there to be executed is a different question.

Not to deviate from plausible truth, one necessary execution was the creation of a leadership role for the newly formed biomolecules. Why is a leader required? A leader directs the actions of others. In this context, the compendium of diverse biomolecules need direction.

The other emergent need was sustenance. Biomolecules needed to remain in form to retain their identities, otherwise, they would be ripped apart and would be lost or recycled. Perhaps this survival need is rooted deep in the nature of matter. Even inside life systems, all forms of biomolecules have a fixed life span before they are turned over and recycled. This strange phenomenon is seen in living systems. Even the same molecules outside of life systems decay. Then what is the difference between biomolecules inside and outside life systems? The difference is that the molecules that die inside life systems are replaced. This does not happen outside of living systems.

Richard Dawkins said in his book that genes survive selfishly. They tend to preserve themselves. He proposed that it is the gene that survives and evolves—not the organism as evolutionary theory proposes. This book was a bestseller—a testament to the public accepting this bizarre idea.

The basic proposal is that genes have a molecular way of replicating themselves and surviving against competition (possibly from other genes). I have not heard hue and cry about this outlandish idea. This means many people believe it. This is surprising because the main tenet of evolutionary theory is that there is no plan or purpose to life system evolution. It is supposed to be a random, undirected process.

What happened in the earth's primordial soup was that evolving molecules, especially nucleic acids, directed processes facilitating the formation of replicating units. Whether you accept or struggle to understand this view does not matter. That is what happened. Gene-directed processes replicate and make copies. This is a fundamental step in the origin of life. Life systems copy and propagate themselves. This happens at the individual level and at the species level. This is only possible because our nucleic acid, DNA, has molecular programs etched in them that allow replication.

Note that the process of replication and propagation is carried out in diverse ways in modern life systems we see today:

both prokaryotic and eukaryotic. The mechanisms of replication are far more diverse in viruses and other selfish gene elements than in other life systems. The point I make is not the diversity in mechanisms of replication but the fact that there is always a role for proteins in this process that assists nucleic acids. Proteins were the executors while nucleic acids provided the instruction codes.

The kinds of proteins we talk about are the enzymes involved in DNA or RNA replication. In modern day organisms, there are many proteins binding to the DNA. They are collectively called DNA-binding proteins and have a variety of roles to play in keeping the DNA or RNA in the functional state.

Histones are one such class of proteins. There are many types of histones too. They help roll DNA strands like a thread coiled around a spindle. They also determine the access to regions of DNA for deciphering the codes. DNA polymerase is another protein that plays the role of deciphering the DNA codes for the purpose of making copies.

RNA polymerase is an enzyme that deciphers the DNA codes for the purpose of making proteins. Physically, DNA or RNA are thread-like structures that remain coiled in the resting state. To access them, they need to be uncoiled. This requires the action of another enzyme called Helicase. There are other proteins acting as chaperones guiding DNA-deciphering enzymes to precise locations within the DNA.

My objective is to illustrate the point that several proteins are required for the genes to work. These proteins evolved in the primordial soup just as the genes did. There must have been a lot of coevolution of these proteins and DNA or RNA. Theorists on the origin of life claim RNA appeared first in this primordial soup. At first, this was an RNA world. DNA probably had not yet formed. Then the RNA formed molecular alliances with the proteins, and it was RNA-protein world. At some point later, the DNA must have emerged and so on.

Whether it was RNA or DNA that formed first is not a problem for us. What is important is to know is: when RNA or DNA started encoding information. In other words, when did they form genes? This is like writing a computer program. Use of the purine and pyrimidine alphabets (just like 0 and 1 used in computer languages) in various sequences happening randomly nature was able to encode executable commands.

In biological parlance, this is called genetic influence.

Those who wonder how randomly arranged sequences of bases can encode information and how they direct the biological theater are advised to read about basic biology. Incredible as it seems, that is what happens in nature. The same sense of wonderment occurs when you see invisible computer binary programs perform miraculous tasks in your electronic devices. You never question how 0s and 1s in sequences worked, but you are quick to question when bases in DNA and RNA do the same.

You can write sentences by combining letters in different, but pre-defined or predictable sequences that conform to the language rules. The sentence meaning emerges but is still abstract. You can write a sentence, like: "I want an apple," but an apple will not get up and walk to you. Action requires an executor to carry out the task.

There are thousands of books and journals filled with all kinds of information. They are of no use if nobody reads and comprehends them before acting. For many years, we have studied in schools and colleges to comprehend the information in technical books. Then we become capable of performing useful tasks. We become the executors.

DNA or RNA is like a book containing biological information about life tasks. But the DNA or RNA cannot accomplish these tasks by themselves. They need the proteins to execute their orders. The fun part is these executors are themselves coded by DNA or RNA. That means nucleic acids (DNA or RNA) have the power to create information and create their own workforce to do what they want.

It may sound difficult to believe. It might even sound like science-fiction. How can lifeless, brainless molecules bring about the Show of Life that has been running non-stop for over 3.5 billion years? It is such a successful blockbuster show with many actors—with something like 30 million known lifeforms.

There may be many millions of other actors about whom we know nothing.

It is difficult to believe that spontaneously evolved RNA or DNA in early earth's pre-biotic soup orchestrated the greatest show in the Universe where they write the script and take care of the casting and the direction as well.

RNA formed as the early nucleic acid blueprint for life. It programmed the design of proteins, forming the RNA-Protein world. These RNA and protein molecules formed the early genes which survived. This is the tenet of the hypothesis of selfish genes. These early genes formed links with other genes—becoming bigger. Or they exchanged genes with other gene groups.

There was a battle for supremacy.

There were surely attempts to encroach on other spaces as well as rob the genes, a legacy that continues to this day in the form of selfish gene elements like viruses.

The laws of genetic inheritance tell us that genes get passed down through the generations. This is called vertical gene transfer. But, in the pre-biotic soup, this transfer of genes happened more by horizontal transfer between entities. To this day this sort of horizontal gene transfer happens a lot between microbes and even between microbes and man. In the case of the latter, the form of retroviruses is like the AIDS virus. A good example is antibiotic resistance gene transfer between microbes.

Going back to the pre-biotic era, when no lifeforms existed, genes ruled the world. They were newly formed molecular associations gaining informational content. The emergence of information led to the ability to control the matter around it.

One foremost event leading to compartmentalized life forms was the origin of enclosures around the genes and proteins called cell membranes which politically speaking is the border between lifeforms. There was a lot of border control happening. Every primitive lifeform tried to protect its genes. If Dawkins is right, it is the other way round. It was the gene providing protection and surviving. The cell membrane was craftily executed.

In diverse viruses infecting bacteria, archaea and eukaryotes, numerous different capsid proteins exist but the idea of enclosing the selfish gene is still the same. It is equally true that capsid-less viruses exist for each of the major classes of viruses. So, the evolution of microbes, especially viruses which possibly were the earliest precursors of life systems, went both ways: capsid-covered and capsid-less.

The history of life is a story of coevolution of selfish gene elements and their cellular hosts, says Eugene Koonin from National Institutes of Health, US. This coevolution is often referred to as an arms race. Cellular life forms evolved ways, often multi-layered defenses, of protecting themselves from invasion of foreign genetic material. Going with the theme of selfish gene elements trying to survive at the cost of others, this phenomenon is as old as the origin of life itself.

The strategic decision taken by cells makes them either fight or flight. Cells decide to fight an invading genetic element or commit suicide. Biologists call this programmed cell death. The cells activate their program of induced cell death when the foreign gene stress exceeds manageable limits. This has a purpose. By doing so, dead cells make it difficult for the invaded gene element to survive and thereby limit its propagation.

Ultimately, viruses like the Corona virus could be involved in establishing their gene supremacy just like the scores of other microbes out there in nature. I raised the question many times throughout this book.

What is the objective of this tiny virus when it infects man?

I said the Corona virus is not interested in your money, wealth or land. But they may be keen to spread their genes. This is a strange idea, but worth considering. This continuing battle for gene supremacy has happened since the origin of life itself.

The Corona virus gained unworthy attention from Homo sapiens for unknown reasons. I argue that social media had a greater role to play here than any biology. But there are classes of viruses like the Retroviruses which, as I said earlier, occupy 8% of human gene territory. This means something. Bizarrely, they have an 8% market share of human gene operations. Why should the retrovirus occupy the human genes to this level? What business have they here? How much market share they own in other life forms needs to be looked at to conclude how successful they have been in the genetic arms race.

What is the status of utilization and control of atomic matter? Microbes gained control of atomic matter on the planet. We humans have ownership of only 0.5% of the global biomass. Microbes own 800 times more bio-matter than us. We are a small minority of shareholders who would not even be invited to the shareholder meeting.

I feel that microbes constantly and quickly find solutions to planetary problems using their gene technologies. Compared to us, they are more adept at inventing new solutions. They crafted so many things on Earth that we can only look at in absolute awe. I described many microbial wonders in different parts of this book. We humans are beneficiaries of microbial designs. We should not complain too much about an occasional pandemic.

The consequences of pandemic overreaction are our problem.

From a biologic point of view, there is an ongoing evolution of the man-microbe relationship. I'm not sure there will ever be an end to this drama. This could be a show that goes on until the end of time. Because microbes evolve so quickly, by the time man's body catches up, it is forced to learn new ways of adapting to an emergent microbe or variant. We will be busy forever—that is the nature of the life game.

Comfort can be taken from realizing we humans are small players in the grand scheme of things happening on our planet.

Be assured.

Nature knows what is good and what needs to be done.

.